I0540280

The New Old: Crafting Your Best Later Life

By

Erika Andersen

The New Old:
Crafting Your Best Later Life

Copyright © Erika Andersen (2025)

All rights reserved. No part of this publication may be reproduced, stored in a retrieval system, or transmitted, in any form or by any means, without the prior written permission of the publisher.

Paperback ISBN: 979-8-89576-079-6
Hardback ISBN: 979-8-89576-080-2

Published by:
Belenos Books

Praise for The New Old.

"With The New Old, Erika Andersen offers a refreshing, empowering approach to creating 'later lives' that perfectly reflect who we've become, and who we want to be; our third acts."

—Sari Botton, Editor Oldster Magazine, and author of the memoir And You May Find Yourself...Confessions of a Late-Blooming Gen-X Weirdo.

"In The New Old, Erika Andersen gives retirement a makeover – and hands you the tools to design and live a third act that's meaningful, joyful, and uniquely yours."

—Bonnie Hammer, Former Vice Chair NBC Universal, author and businesswoman

"Retirement used to be seen as a slow slide into irrelevant old age. In The New Old, Erika Andersen encourages you to break that paradigm and create a meaningful and uplifting third act for your life."

—Danny Meyer, Founder and Executive Chairman, Union Square Hospitality Group

"Unlike all the books that give specific advice for old age - what to eat, how to save, where to live - Erika Andersen has done something different: she offers a way to design the later life you want, and the skills and mindset to achieve it. It's honest, friendly, and practical - I found The New Old fun to read and very useful."

—Kathy Dore, Media industry innovator and retired executive

"Even if you're not ready to retire, The New Old offers a practical approach to creating your best 'second half.' Erika's guidance is inspiring, warm and honest."

    —Benita Fitzgerald Mosley, Olympic Gold Medalist and
      Non-Profit CEO

"The New Old is a wonderful support for the second half of life. Reading Erika Andersen is like having a wise friend who points you toward vitality and purpose."

    —Lorraine C. Ladish, author of Tu Mejor Edad and CEO and
      founder of VivaFifty!

"If you want to custom design a later life that works best for you, The New Old is a fantastic resource. I'm excited to put it into practice.

    —David Kline, Former President Spectrum Reach and
      EVP Charter Communications

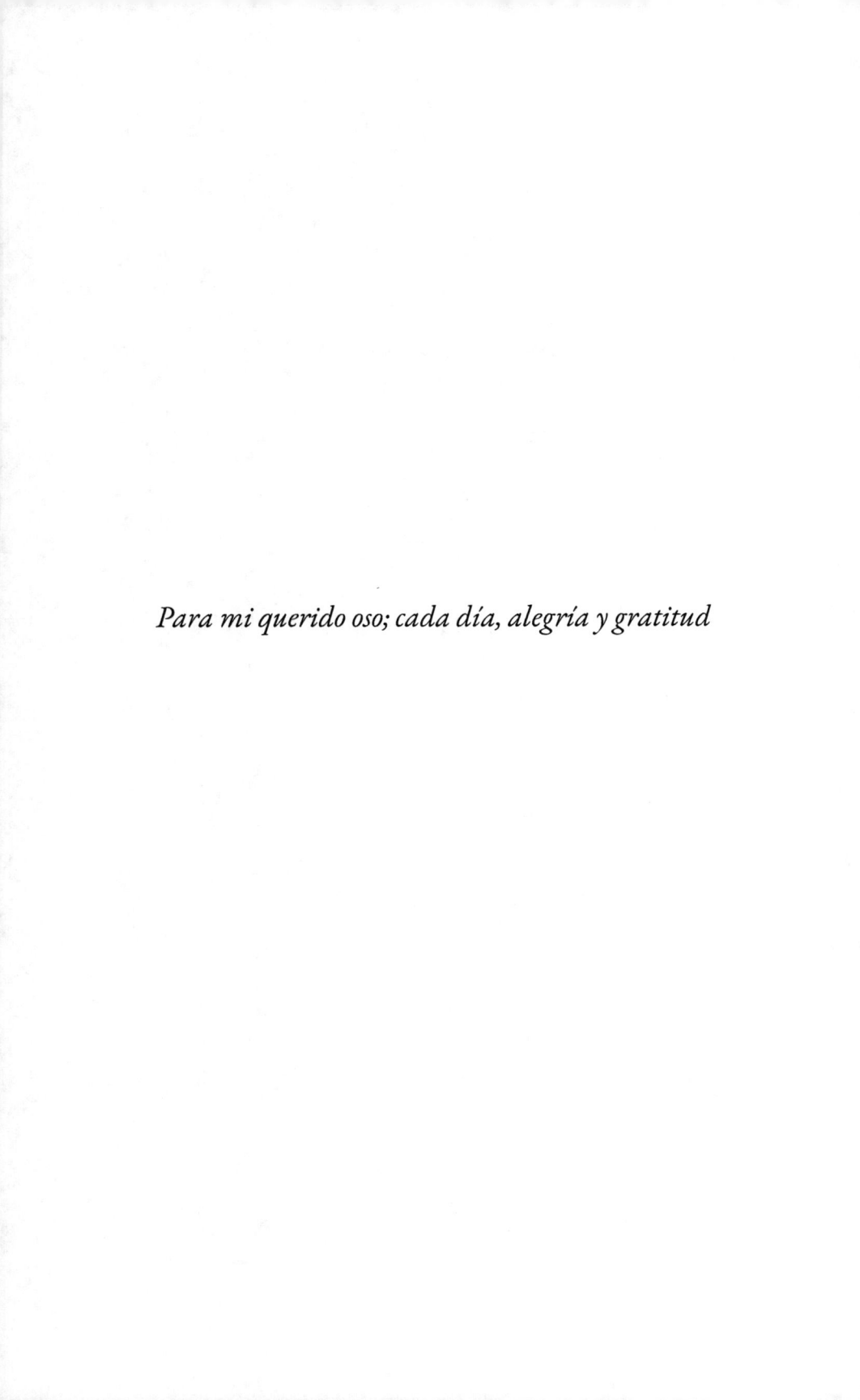

Para mi querido oso; cada día, alegría y gratitud

Table of Contents

1. Why This Book, and Why Now

We human beings don't have much experience of being old. Just a hundred years ago, a person's chances of living to be 65 were pretty slim. Even if you were lucky enough to make that golden number, you could only expect to live to be 75 or, with great good fortune, 80.

In contrast, the vast majority of people alive today will reach their 65th birthday. What's more, today's reasonably healthy, non-smoking 65-year-old has about even odds of living to 90.[1] Put another way: in 1920, less than 1 in 20 people were over 65. Now, in the developed world, the figure is 1 in 6.

That's why I've called this book "The New Old." This reality of most people living into their 70s, 80s and 90s is indeed new. Until now, a life generally had two chapters and an epilogue. Chapter I: Be born, grow up, and become an adult; the first 20-25 years. Chapter 2: Create a family and a career and find your place in the world; the next 35-40 years. Epilogue: Step back from the world and drift into a twilight of increasing frailty and dependence; 5-15 years, if you were lucky.

And as being old has become increasingly common, we're starting to see that we're still largely operating in the two-chapters-and-an-epilogue mode: we don't have much of a roadmap for what a full, vital, third chapter should or could look like. It's as though we've all been driving down a well-marked highway, and now, post-65, we're having to go off-road, without even a GPS.

We have some vague notions about retirement and not having to work every day; we all know we should be thinking about how to make our money last if we're not working for pay; we hope our life will include a community of family and friends; perhaps we're thinking about what we might be doing if we're not doing what we've always done...

In other words, most of us are not very clear about what those last decades of our life will be like.

As I walk into my seventies, this has become—as you might imagine—much more personal and real for me. To prepare to write this book, I've had dozens of conversations with clients, colleagues, friends and family members who are also in the latter part of their lives, and I've found that many of them have similar questions. What does it mean to be old? How is it different from being young? What do I want to do and what will I be able to do? Others, I've noticed, are simply avoiding the whole subject and just plowing ahead, business as usual (we'll talk later about the downsides of that).

I've also read lots of articles and books (we baby boomers are writing about aging with a vengeance these days). I've noticed that most of the books being written about aging focus on giving specific advice about the practical aspects (how to save and budget, where to live, whether to downsize), the physical aspects (what to eat, how to stay fit, which supplements to take), or the medical realities (dealing with doctors, living with illness, extending your life through various means).

However, I'm looking at this situation through the lens of the work I've done over the past 40 years, helping people and organizations get clear about the future they want to create for themselves, and how to achieve it. Given that lens, it's not surprising that I've noticed the absence of a handbook for taking a step back and thinking about this whole third act of your life in a more intentional and holistic way. In an earlier book, *Being Strategic*, I defined the idea of being strategic as "consistently making the core directional efforts that will best move you toward your hoped-for future." I'm offering this book as a guide to doing just that: getting clearer about your "hoped-for future" in this latter part of your life and creating your own roadmap for getting there.

I'm making some assumptions about who you are, as well. I imagine you're someone in your 50s, 60s, or beyond who is starting to see that you aren't as clear as you want to be about the rest of your life. For the past 30 or 40 years, you've focused on family, career, and financial security. But now your kids, if you have them, are grown; you're starting to understand that you don't want to (or can't) work the same way you did when you were younger. However, you don't want to just drift into an old age of feeling invisible and ineffectual. You want to be an active creator of your later life. If that's a pretty good description of you, I think you'll find this conversation valuable. Let's get started.

---

[1] Kiburz, S. (2024). *Chart of the day: Odds to live at age 65.* Crews Bank and Trust. https://www.crews.bank/charts/odds-to-live-at-age-65

2. Approaching This Third Act

"Aging is not lost youth, but a new stage of opportunity and strength." —Betty Friedan

When I write a book, I'm always trying to crack a code for my readers, to find a simple, practical approach to a complex topic. The idea of finding and sharing key principles for addressing important problems has always appealed to me.

In 1990, I read a book called *The Fifth Discipline*[1] that was very much aligned with and supportive of this approach, and it had a profound effect on me: it was my first exposure to someone else talking about this way of approaching life and challenges. Peter Senge, the book's author, described this kind of thinking as looking at an entire system and finding the few key points that, if you can affect them, will have the highest positive impact on the whole system.

That's a perfect summary of what I've tried to do in all my writing and teaching: to find the key principles, models, or frameworks that will allow the reader to have the greatest positive impact on their "system." In previous books, the systems I've focused on have been leadership, learning and change. In this book, the system we're focusing on is old age, and the code I'm trying to help you crack is how to craft your best later life. In the service of that, I'd like to offer you three key principles that we'll use throughout the book as our framework for addressing this "system" of old age:

Principle I: Be the Boss of Your Life

As I've spoken to people in their 60s and beyond, one complaint I hear over and over is that they feel "invisible." When I dig into this and ask what they mean, most respond that they feel others are ignoring them, making decisions for them, or assuming they will be OK doing what those others tell them to do. For example, I've heard stories of grown children trying to make major decisions for their parents–about medical care, housing, or finances–without including their parents in the discussion. People have told me about conversations where their professional expertise has been ignored or dismissed in favor of the input of younger colleagues, even when they express the same ideas. In other words, "invisible" is another way of saying "powerless."

Unfortunately, this is not simply an individual problem; much of society has negative cultural attitudes about older people and about the process of aging.[2] And these attitudes, these beliefs and feelings underlie and reinforce these ways of behaving toward us that tend to disempower and disenfranchise us as older adults.

Studies have shown that older people are often depicted as weak, unattractive, and senile. Other cultural stereotypes portray us as frail, feeble, financially distressed, and not contributing to society.[3] And these stereotypes persist, even though the majority of people in their later years are competent, healthy, and independent. These attitudes have come to be called ageism, and some researchers have called it "the last socially acceptable prejudice."[4] One of the reasons it's so pervasive is that it often masquerades as "care"–as in, "I'm not disempowering my mom, I'm just 'taking care' of her." These stereotypes are also, unfortunately, reinforced because they contain a grain of truth: there are, in fact, some fragile, dependent, unhealthy old people, and so we all get painted with that brush.

No wonder we can feel powerless; it's hard not to be affected by these pervasive stereotypes, especially when we see and hear them in the media and from those around us on a daily basis.

That's why it's so important in this third chapter of life to establish your own sense of who you are and to take charge of your circumstances: to be the boss of your life. Being the boss of your life is a powerful antidote to society's limiting and limited expectations of old people. Now, one caveat: in using the word "boss," I'm not implying that you can have total control over the process of getting old; just that you can have a clear sense of yourself and how you want to live your life, work to make that happen, and be proactive in your response when the unexpected occurs (as it surely will).

I've noted a related phenomenon in my work in organizations over the past four decades. People who take full responsibility for their own job and for their success or failure in it tend to be seen by others as more mature, more powerful, more reliable–and they are treated differently by others than those who assume that they don't have power in their job and will be controlled by others. I've seen this phenomenon at every job level, from newly hired assistant to CEO.

Over the past few years, I've noticed the same dynamic at play with older friends and colleagues –and with myself–with regard to how we're living our lives. When we assume, as older adults, that we have agency, that it's our prerogative to decide what's best for us and how to achieve it, and then to act toward those ends, others respond by treating us with more respect. They ask our opinion, include us in decisions, listen to our point of view, and cede power to us in situations that affect us and over which we should have control.

So how can you be the boss of this third chapter of your life? How do you avoid falling prey to society's (and perhaps your own) expectations of dependence and frailty? We'll focus on three practical ways to "be the boss":

-*Keep envisioning your future*: Good bosses in organizations create and keep moving toward a clear vision of the future for their department or company. Bosses who operate like this tend to get the best results, and they—and those who work with and for them—seem to have the most enjoyable journey along the way.

I've seen that this is true of individuals, as well; those who aren't "bosses" in the traditional sense. Generally speaking, I've noticed that those people who are clear about what's important to them and consistent in making an effort to achieve it tend to have the most satisfying lives. To reiterate the definition of being strategic I mentioned earlier: they "consistently make the core directional efforts that will best move them toward their hoped-for future." They get and stay clear about the future they want to create for themselves and focus their energies on making that future a reality.

However, even if you've been good at doing this in the middle of your life, it's easy to stop doing it when you get older. Too often, when we're no longer focused on advancing our careers or raising our kids, we can start to drift. We can assume that we've achieved all our big goals and that the rest is just repeats and slow decline, and we can wander into living a less intentional life. Sadly, others can see and feel this—and they're all too happy to step in and start running our lives for us.

In this chapter, I'll teach you how to create a future vision that clarifies what you most want from this part of your life, and that is flexible enough to change as your life and the lives of your loved ones evolve.

-*Make it Happen*: Good bosses don't stop at creating a vision; they make sure it gets implemented. This is where envisioning your future gets practical. Once you've decided who you want to be and how you want your later life to look and feel, how will you make it a reality? We'll start on the level of intention: you'll create a handful of intentions, core statements about how you intend to fulfill your vision. I'll help you make sure that your intentions have a good ROE (Return on Effort); that they'll be powerfully helpful to you in achieving your hoped-for future. Then, we'll talk about translating your intentions into actions and how to make it more likely that you'll actually take those steps.

-*Lead Your Crew*: The older we get, the more we tend to accumulate people around us who help us and support our success. As our physical condition gets more complicated, even if we're basically healthy, we acquire doctors, nurses, physical therapists. We also gather people who help us with the tasks of daily life; perhaps those who clean our house, take care of our pets, or fix our plumbing. They're often people we hire, but they can also be friends or family members. For example, my son and my sons-in-law are a lot stronger than either my husband or me at this point, and I'm happy to have them move and carry stuff when they're around.

But when these people are professionals—and maybe most especially when they're medical professionals—we can tend to think of them as our bosses, rather than as part of a group of supporters of whom *we're* the boss. In this chapter, I'll share practical approaches for creating a support system with those who provide services to you: people who are collaborative and supportive, but with you firmly in the driver's seat. We'll talk about the importance of communicating your vision and making sure you have understanding and buy-in from those who are most critical to its success. We'll also talk about the power of delegating and how to do it well, and we'll look at how to ensure that you have the best resources to help you make critical decisions. Finally, we'll talk about holding yourself and others accountable to manifesting what you've envisioned and agreed to, and the difficult task of asking people to leave your crew when they're not serving your best interests.

Principle II: Master Your Mindset

A fascinating study came out of the Yale School of Public Health about 20 years ago.[5] They asked 638 people, men and women in their 50s and

60s, questions to determine their perceptions about aging. Then, they followed this group for 23 years. They found that those who had more positive perceptions of aging (for example, who disagreed with the statement "as you get older, you are less useful") lived on average 7.6 years longer–and that's after controlling for factors such as age, gender, socioeconomic status, functional health, self-reported health, and loneliness.

Let's reflect on this for a moment. That means that simply having a more hopeful and positive mindset about aging yielded bigger longevity benefits than all the physical efforts about which we hear so much: better results than quitting smoking, losing weight, exercising regularly, or lowering your cholesterol or blood pressure. Doing any of those things, it turns out, will generally add 1 to 4 years to your life.

But having a consistently more positive mindset about getting old? *7.6 more years.*

And that study was only the first of its kind. Many subsequent studies have shown even stronger correlations. One study of 14,000 older adults from the Harvard School of Public Health in 2022[6] found that those most satisfied with aging had a 43% lower risk of dying from any cause over the 4 years of the study than those with more negative perceptions. That is, they were about half as likely to die, period.

I love this. I've been encouraging–and teaching–people to master their mindset for 40 years, and I've often opined that learning to do so may be the single most powerful capability we can develop as humans. So, you can imagine how thrilled I am to have found all this evidence about the power of mindset when it comes to aging!

Think of it this way: there are many things we can't control as we get older. We may be subject to all kinds of difficult physical and emotional realities–hereditary conditions, diseases, accidents, deaths of loved ones and friends, and other losses. But this extraordinarily powerful tool to improve our later lives is entirely within our control. We can master how we think about aging and about ourselves as older adults.

Here's how we'll approach developing this critical capability:

-Learn to Manage your Self-talk: Our beliefs–about ourselves and others, about the world around us, about aging and dying–show up in how we talk to ourselves. You know that you talk to yourself, right? Almost all of us do: it's like a silent mental monologue that runs, mostly just underneath our conscious awareness, all the time. Often, it's pretty benign (*hot day I like that girl's shoes wonder what I should make for dinner when will they finish building those apartments did I remember to get Advil...*), and we generally just ignore it.

Unfortunately, it can also be the opposite of benign. That voice can say things to us that have a powerful negative impact on the quality and, as it turns out per those studies, the quantity of our lives. We can tell ourselves, for instance, that we're incapable or unlovable. We can tell ourselves as older people that we are (or will become) useless, frail, "out of it," dependent, unhealthy...and on and on.

The very good news is that you can learn to manage this self-talk. We can recognize any unhelpful self-talk we might have about aging and revise it to be more supportive of a healthy, productive and joyful later life. I'll teach you the skill, we'll practice, and you'll think about how to apply your new skills of managing your self-talk for the best outcomes in your own life.

- Become More Present: You may have heard the word "mindfulness" more and more over the past decade. Though people talk about it as though it's a complex and esoteric practice, it's actually very simple: it means focusing one's attention on what's taking place in the present moment without judgement.

It's simple, but it's not necessarily easy. One of the problems with the mental monologue we talked about earlier is that it distracts us from experiencing the moment we're in. Much of our internal "chatter" is about the past, the future, and about things that have never happened and never will happen. Not only do we get pulled into thinking about all these non-existent things, we often have strong feelings about them. For example, how many times have you gone over and over in your head a conversation that you wish you had had with someone where you tell them exactly what you think of them in the most eloquent way? And as you're having that made-up conversation in your head, you're getting madder and madder at the person because you didn't say those things that, in your head, you were able to say so perfectly, and then you start thinking about that person, and things they've done to you in the past that made you angry at them, and how you're right and they're wrong and....

That's the opposite of mindfulness.

It turns out that learning to focus your attention on the present moment is not only good for you, it feels wonderful, as well. Study after study shows that increased mindfulness has both psychological and physiological benefits.[7] Becoming more present can also help you manage your self-talk: a great deal of our negative self-talk is focused on things that don't actually exist (negative predictions, unlikely outcomes, fantasies about what others are thinking or doing relative to us), and when you're more focused on noticing what does exist, that fantasy-based self-talk starts to lose its hold on you.

We'll hone this skill in real life: I'll help you to become more present by focusing on the current realities you most love and enjoy, which can become positive magnets for your awareness.

-*Cultivate Gratitude*: Gratitude is my favorite emotion. I love the way it feels to be grateful. And it seems that I'm not alone; in study after study, feeling and expressing gratitude has been shown to make people both happier and healthier.[8]

The very good news is that these studies also show that it's relatively simple and straightforward to develop a daily gratitude practice. In other words, you can become more grateful. And guess what–becoming more grateful relies on (and develops) two mental skills: mastering your self-talk and becoming more present. We'll take advantage of this synergy among the three skills to build mindset mastery as a key element of your getting-old-well toolkit.

Principle III: Get Good at Change

The last book I wrote before this one was called *Change from the Inside Out*, and it's about how the world and our lives are changing faster than ever before, why it's hard, and how to get better at moving with and through change.

It's targeted primarily to leaders in organizations, but the skills and approaches I outline are universally applicable. And even as I was writing it (since I was already in my late 60s), I was reflecting on how much change there is in getting old. Our bodies, our minds, our relationships, our approach to work and leisure–almost every aspect of our lives changes a lot from 60 to 70 to 80 and beyond. I notice that it's also often the hardest kind of change: change that's imposed upon us rather than change we initiate. And, to make it even more challenging, society often implies the opposite: that once you're past your "productive years" and into "old age," it's all kind of the same; boring and unchanging.

A funny but poignant example: recently, I found an article in one of the most widely-read US newspapers about "how to assess your fitness at any age." It was a well-designed interactive online article that offered 5 self-tests you could take and then note your results to see how you stacked up against your age peers. The only problem? The age categories were 20-30, 30-40, 40-50, 50-60, and then 60+. When I took the tests, it told me my results were above average for "women in my age group," implying that the same result would be above average for a woman of 62, 75, 83, or...100? Seems ridiculous, right? In fact, I've found that my physical condition is changing more quickly now than when I was younger. For instance, I'd say that my results wouldn't have been much different when I was 43 than when I was 30–but my results now, at 73, are definitely different than they would have been at 60. I'm fortunate to be in very good health, but I notice that my strength, balance, and flexibility are all somewhat less than they were 10 or 15 years ago. It's not terrible, and I'm working on it–but it's a change.

As I've talked with others in this latter part of life, many have noted another factor that makes change even more challenging now; our tendency, as older people, to want to settle into routines and to resist and denigrate "the new." One friend of mine said to me recently, "Sometimes I feel like a parody of an old person–I actually find myself saying things like 'why, in my day we never would have acted like that,' or 'every time they update my phone, I can't do something I'm used to doing.' It's embarrassing to see how I'm getting set in my ways."

So, I propose to you that, as older people, if we want to thrive through our changing lives in this changing world, it behooves us to go in the opposite direction; to become even better at changing than our younger counterparts. Now, another caveat: I'm not proposing that routines or sameness are bad. In fact, I've found (and many of my interviewees have told me) that having pleasant and healthy daily routines as you age is a lovely and comfortable counterbalance to all the changes you'll encounter. In the best case, our routines can create a kind of ballast that grounds us as we move through change.

I'm going to offer you three approaches for becoming more change-capable:

- ***Understand How We Go Through Change***: I wrote *Change from the Inside Out* to share the understanding and approaches my colleagues and I at Proteus have developed and use to help leaders and organizations go through transformations large and small in their professional lives. But, as I noted earlier, the core skills and insights I outlined are completely applicable to this journey of older age. The element I think you'll find most useful is what we've come to call "The Change Arc": it describes what happens, psychologically and emotionally, when an individual successfully goes through a change. I'll explain it and help you build the necessary skills to move through the Arc more quickly and easily when you're facing any change. In other words, we'll build your "change muscles."

- ***Modify Gracefully***: One of the many problems with that "how to stay fit at any age" article I mentioned was that it proposed no modifications of any kind to the physical tasks suggested. For example, one of the tests involved doing "burpees." As you may know, this exercise involves squatting, thrusting your legs backward in a jumping motion to a plank position, doing a full push-up, jumping your legs back to a squat position, and then quickly standing upright. It's a very good conditioning exercise–but only if you don't have problems with your knees, hips, or shoulders. Even if you don't have specific problems, for most older people, it puts a lot of unnecessary stress on those joints; there are better ways to get the same conditioning without the stress.

Learning to modify various aspects of your life as you get older is a key part of the change capability necessary to having a great later life. This skill consists of being able to recognize when something needs modifying (from your exercise routine, to how you approach work, to eating habits, to relationships, to medical support); figuring out how to modify it in a way and to an extent that works for you; getting whatever support or agreement you need from others (back to leading your crew); and then making the modification without giving yourself a hard time about it (back to mastering your self-talk).

In this part of our conversation, you'll learn how to become a master of graceful modification and then decide where you may need to apply your skills right now.

-Discover and Explore–Anything: Until fairly recently, scientists thought that cognitive decline in older adults was an inevitable part of aging. But multiple studies done over the past few decades have shown that most people's mental abilities don't decline with age *unless they stop using them.*[9] The italics are mine because I find this so critically important: our ability to learn, grow, and develop as older people is a strictly use it or lose it proposition, and therefore there's no reason to assume that we can't acquire new skills, knowledge, and ability at any age.

For me, that's one of the coolest things about getting old: since my kids are grown and I'm spending less time working, I now have lots of bandwidth to explore new things. For instance (and I'm sure this will come up often as an example), my husband and I now spend most of our time living in the north of Spain. Having spent the previous 70+ years living in the US, it's hugely engaging, challenging, and fun to spend my days learning a new language, a new culture, a new city, and all that that entails. Every day, I wonder about a hundred things, ask a dozen questions, acquire new ways to think and operate. I can almost feel new synapses forming!

In this part of the book, I'll share a model from another of my books, *Be Bad First*, that will support your efforts to learn and discover, and we'll refer back to your future vision to select areas for learning that will be particularly fun and meaningful for you.

A Thread That Runs Through Everything

There's one more element of a great later life that informs and impacts all three of these principles, and we'll talk about it as a final element: connection with other people. It turns out that human connection is even more important as we age than in our earlier lives, and that in many Western countries, there's an epidemic of loneliness among older people. Loneliness and social isolation represent significant risk factors for both physical and psychological well-being as we age.[10] Many older people lose their partners through divorce or death, and they may become distant from family and friends because of geography, changing priorities, or estrangement of various kinds. And often, as old people, we've lost the knack of creating new relationships and don't have the environments we had previously (work or family commitments) that made it easier to connect with others.

You may feel that you have all the close relationships you need in this part of your life, and if so, consider yourself fortunate. But, if not, we'll leverage the skills you've learned throughout the book (especially for managing your self-talk and learning new things) to help you create new relationships and connections that will enrich and enliven your later life and support you in creating the life you've envisioned.

And Finally...

As an example, I'll bring you into the life that my husband and I are creating for ourselves in our 70s so you can see how we're manifesting our later life vision. And as my final gift to you, I'll share a "quick start guide" for crafting your best later life, in case you need a jump-start for using all these skills and approaches.

Making it Practical, Starting Now

As I said earlier, whenever I write a book, I focus on offering practical, simple, fundamental ways to help my readers solve a key problem. So, before we go on, let's do a bit of self-reflection: I want to give you a chance to see where you're starting from in these skills and attitudes we'll be covering. As you take this quiz, remember that the goal is not to "get a good score" but rather to be accurate about your current starting point. Then, when you finish the book, you can come back and re-assess: I hope that the skills and insights you develop in the course of our journey together will have improved your ability to create the later life you most want.

For each question below, note what's true for you now on a scale of 1-5, with 1 being "not at all," 3 being "somewhat" and 5 being "very much so" (you'll also find the quiz at thenewoldbook.com, where you can note your score and save it to come back to later).

I'm clear about what I want my later life to be like.	
I'm confident I can create the future I want.	
I know what to do to make my hoped-for future happen.	
I can make tough decisions as needed to have the life I want.	
I have the people around me I need to support my later life.	
I have clear agreements with the people in my life.	
I talk to myself in accurate and helpful ways.	
I can shift my mental monologue when it doesn't support me.	
I can focus on and appreciate the present moment.	
I refocus my mind on the present when I get caught in negative thinking.	

I feel grateful for many things in my life.	
I practice gratitude every day.	
I know how people go through change.	
I'm good at moving through unexpected changes.	
I recognize when I need to modify some aspect of my life.	
I modify as needed without resentment.	
I explore new things on a regular basis.	
I'm confident in my ability to learn and grow throughout my life.	
I have human connections that support and enrich my daily experience.	
I know how to create healthy new relationships.	

Now that you have a sense of where you're starting from, I have one more important thing to share with you before you decide what you want to create....

---

[1] Senge, P. M. (2006). The fifth discipline: The art and practice of the learning organization. Deckle Edge

[2] WHO. (2016). *Discrimination and negative attitudes about ageing are bad for your health.* World Health Organization. https://www.who.int/news/item/29-09-2016-discrimination-and-negative-attitudes-about-ageing-are-bad-for-your-health

[3] Blakeborough, D. (2008). "Old people are useless": Representations of aging on The Simpsons. *Canadian Journal on Aging/La revue canadienne du vieillissement, 27*(1), 57-67. https://www.cambridge.org/core/journals/canadian-journal-on-aging-la-revue-canadienne-du-vieillissement/article/abs/old-people-are-useless-representations-of-aging-on-the-simpsons/C2231100E1D799401938FA98EA8A212A

[4] Weir, K. (2023). Ageism is one of the last socially acceptable prejudices. Psychologists are working to change that. American Psychological Association. https://www.apa.org/monitor/2023/03/cover-new-concept-of-aging

[5] Yale News. (2002). Thinking Positively About Aging Extends Life More Than Exercise and Not Smoking. https://news.yale.edu/2002/07/29/thinking-positively-about-aging-extends-life-more-exercise-and-not-smoking

[6] Harvard T.C. Chan School of Public Health. (2022). *Positive attitude about aging could boost health.* https://www.hsph.harvard.edu/news/hsph-in-the-news/positive-attitude-about-aging-could-boost-health/

[7] Keng, S. L., Smoski, M. J., & Robins, C. J. (2011). Effects of mindfulness on psychological health: A review of empirical studies. *Clinical psychology review, 31*(6), 1041-1056. https://pmc.ncbi.nlm.nih.gov/articles/PMC3679190/#:~:text=Overall%2C%20evidence%20from%20correlational%20research,of%20negative%20affect%20and%20psychopathological

[8] Harvard Medical School. (2021). Giving Thanks Can Make You Happier. Harvard Health Publishing. https://www.health.harvard.edu/healthbeat/giving-thanks-can-make-you-happier#:~:text=In%20positive%20psychology%20research%2C%20gratitude,express%20gratitude%20in%20multiple%20ways.

[9] Wu, R., Church-Lang, J. (2023). *To Stay Sharp As You Age, Learn New Skills.* Scientific American. https://www.scientificamerican.com/article/to-stay-sharp-as-you-age-learn-new-skills/

[10] Valtorta, N., & Hanratty, B. (2012). Loneliness, isolation and the health of older adults: do we need a new research agenda?. *Journal of the Royal Society of Medicine, 105*(12), 518-522. https://pmc.ncbi.nlm.nih.gov/articles/PMC3536512/

3. This is a Little Terrifying

"Life is pleasant. Death is peaceful. It's the transition that's troublesome." —Isaac Asimov

You're gonna die. Me too. We're all going to die. And, if you're over 60, you've almost certainly already lived longer than you're going to live from now till the end.

There you have it: the key reason people don't like to think about getting old. At the end of getting old is death.

While researching my previous book on change, I found out that many psychologists believe that fear of the unknown is our deepest fear.[1] And there are so many unknowns in getting old: What will my life be like if I'm not doing the work I've always done, or in the ways I've done it? What will I be like (and, really, who will I be) if I'm not doing that work? How will my relationships change with family, friends, children? What will happen to my health? Will I be able to do the hobbies and activities I've always done–and will I want to? What will the world be like, and will I have a place in it?

And, of course, the biggest unknown: death. Your own death and the deaths of people you love. When will it happen, what will it be like, and can I do anything to delay it or make it less painful?

As we get older, we're surrounded by more and more unknowns, and that scares us. When things scare us, we react in fairly predictable ways–most of them only moderately helpful, at best. You probably remember the core categories of threat response from long-ago psychology classes: fight, flight, and freeze. These ways of responding when we're feeling threatened and afraid can be useful when it comes to physical threat–a saber-tooth tiger chasing us, for instance–but for the more amorphous unknown threats involved in getting old...not so much.

Since we can't literally flee getting old and all the uncertainty it brings, the most common flight reaction I've seen in older people is to avoid the whole topic; to flee mentally, and act as though nothing is changing. I saw one very sad example of this a number of years ago when Sumner Redstone, at that time the chairman and majority stockholder of CBS/Paramount, was forced to relinquish his chairmanship at the age of 92, after a court-ordered examination found that he was suffering from dementia and a severe health-related speech impediment. Redstone had refused to acknowledge that his mental and physical health had deteriorated at all, and still wanted to run the company as though everything were the same, and he was still completely capable.

There was some "fight" in his reaction, as well: fighting against the court's determination of his unfitness and his family's wish for him to step down. I've also seen a lot of day-to-day fighting against fear of the unknown: older people refusing to stop driving, even when doing so is clearly dangerous, or resisting necessary medical advice. And then there's the ultimate "fight" against age: actively refusing to acknowledge the inevitability of death. I just read an article a few weeks ago about a very wealthy middle-aged man focusing all his considerable resources and the vast majority of his time and effort on living in such a way as to never die. I say good luck, but I'm almost sure he'll be disappointed in the end.

And lots of us "freeze" in the face of the unknowns of old age: we get even more change-averse than is the norm for humans of any age, and we try to keep everything in our lives as much the same as possible. We do the same things, watch the same shows, eat the same food, live in the same place, express the same opinions, and rely on the same information. We refuse to expand our habits, our knowledge, our experiences, or perceptions. I believe this functions for many people as a kind of talisman against fear; an elderly version of not stepping on cracks or always having our lucky rabbit's foot.

So, what would be a more useful response to our fear of all the unknowns that surround getting old—particularly the unknown of death?

Confronting Your Fear of the Unknown

I propose a simple response to fear that I have found incredibly helpful throughout my life:

1. **Acknowledge that you are afraid, and then name your fear.**
2. **Note the worst thing that could happen if your fear comes true.**
3. **Ask what you can do to reduce the likelihood of that "worst thing" outcome—or to make it less negative if it's unavoidable (like death).**
4. **Make the necessary plans and do what you've decided.**

So, for example, in my mid-60s, when I started thinking about eventually retiring from work, I began getting anxious about that idea. As soon as I noticed my anxiety, I made the effort to name my fear (step 1). And what I saw after some self-reflection was that I didn't know who I would be if I wasn't working many hours a week as "the founder and CEO of Proteus." I had spent decades with that as a big and important (to me) part of my identity—and the idea of not having that was scary.

I asked myself what was the worst thing that could happen to me in this situation (step 2), and I realized that it was the possibility of not having a clear sense of identity and not having impact or influence, that is, not making any positive difference in the world.

I then thought about how I could make that outcome less likely, and I understood that I needed to clarify what I wanted my post-work identity to be (step 3).

I started by summarizing my curiosity about my later-life identity into a simple question. That question was, "How can I become what comes after the butterfly?" Here's how I came to that: up to that point, I had been thinking of my life as being like the evolution of a caterpillar to a butterfly. I saw my childhood and youth as the caterpillar stage, and it seemed to me that the deeply self-reflective time I spent in a spiritual community in my twenties was "being in the cocoon." I saw being the mother of my children and founder and CEO of my company as my butterfly stage.

However, unlike an actual butterfly, I was now seeing that stage wasn't the end for me: I had to discover and build my next stage of evolution. Creating that curious question–"How can I become what comes after the butterfly?"–helped me move past my fear into finding answers to that question that resonated for me and making plans to help ensure I moved in that direction (step 4).

Then, I began taking action to move toward that new post-butterfly identity, part of which, for me, is writing this book.

So, I encourage you to acknowledge and name your fears about getting old, and then let yourself acknowledge the worst things that could happen if those fears came true. Allow yourself to see and name even the deep, difficult things like, "I will die," "My spouse could die before me," or "I could become physically or mentally incapacitated."

Once you've let yourself see and feel those fears and have said to yourself as honestly as possible what they are (step 1), you can get clear about the worst that could happen relative to them (step 2). Then, you can move through those fears by deciding how to make them less likely or less negative (step 3). Finally, you can plan to do that and take action to implement your plans (step 4).

That's where this book can help. Everything I'm going to share with you here will support you in steps 3 and 4–in getting curious about how to mitigate the impact of the things you fear, selecting approaches that you think will be helpful, and then taking action to do the things you've selected.

So: I intend to support you in responding to your fears of the unknown aspects of aging in helpful, productive ways.

What You Can Do

You, however, have an even more important task ahead of you. You need to be brave enough to face those fears. As Mae West once said, "Getting old is not for the faint of heart." The good news is, the fact that you're still reading and haven't "misplaced" this book into some out-of-the-way nook, never to be found again, proposes to me that you're willing to be brave in this way.

To help you get started, you can use the worksheet below to start facing some of your own personal fears about getting old and deciding how to move through them (you can also find an interactive PDF of this worksheet at thenewoldbook.com):

---

1) What are my three biggest fears about getting old?

a:

b:

---

c:

2) What's the worst thing that could happen regarding each of them?

a:

b:

c:

3) What can I do to make each of those outcomes less likely or less negative?

a:

b:

c:

And if you'd rather just think about this topic vs. writing things down, that's OK too; use whatever approach works for you. I would only encourage you not to avoid doing this work. Think and feel through these issues in some way. Not knowing what scares you most about getting old will make it harder to take best advantage of the rest of this book.

Deep breath.

Let's get started...

---

[1] Carleton, R. N. (2016). Fear of the unknown: One fear to rule them all? *Journal of anxiety disorders, 41,* 5-21.
https://www.sciencedirect.com/science/article/pii/S0887618516300469

Principle I:
Be the Boss of Your Life

4. Keep Envisioning Your Future

*"Aging is an extraordinary process where you become
the person you always should have been."*
—David Bowie

I've noticed for many years that the people I've met who are the most successful tend to have a clear vision of the future they want to create for themselves. Especially when I talk to people in their 30s and 40s who have created lives about which they're mostly pleased and proud, part of the conversation often centers around how happy they are to have been able to achieve the things they hoped for: building a family; doing work that matters to them; establishing strong relationships; having a positive impact on the world.

During the decades when I was coaching senior executives, I saw the same thing. Those who became the most successful had a clear sense of who they wanted to be as leaders and of the enterprise or department they wanted to create. In fact, as their coach, I was often part of the process of their coming to that understanding. When I worked with someone who went from not having a clear sense of their own hoped-for future to having that clear sense, it was sometimes almost magical to see how gaining that clarity changed them. They would become more grounded, more confident, often happier and more enthusiastic. Generally, as soon as they had that vision, they would start wanting to move toward it. Even those around them would comment on the changes they saw in the "envisioner," and I noticed that those who worked for them often started to trust them more and be more willing to work with them to achieve whatever goals they had outlined.

Unfortunately, even those who envision and achieve important and worthwhile goals in the middle of their lives often stop envisioning when they reach their 60s, 70s, or 80s. They may simply clutch on to their former vision: refusing to retire; trying to keep "parenting" their kids or even grandkids, not wanting them to operate as independent beings; or reviewing over and over, to anyone who will listen, their previous moments of glory. Or they might just drift–not doing much, complaining a lot, seeming unhappy with how their later life is unfolding.

In contrast, the older people I've talked to who seem happiest and most contented with their later lives are those who have kept envisioning: who have a clear sense of who they want to be as older people and what they want their later life to be like. Lately, there's been a lot of research that supports this observation of mine. Dan Buettner's *The Blue Zones* (a wonderful book if you haven't read it) found that people who live in the areas of the world with the greatest longevity tend to cultivate a clear sense of purpose[1]. In the Blue Zone of Okinawa, for instance, they call it *ikigai*, usually understood to mean understanding and pursuing a passion or passions and having the feelings of fulfillment and accomplishment that it brings. In Nicoya, Costa Rica, another Blue Zone, seniors talk about having a *plan de vida*, which they define as "why I wake up in the morning." Another study from the National Institutes of Aging further supported the importance of having a clear "why" in later life: people who could articulate a sense of purpose lived up to 7 years longer than those who couldn't.[2]

Let's Get Clear About Our Own Future

I've been using a process to help people and organizations get clear about the future they want to create for themselves for almost 40 years, so I'm going to share with you a version of that same process that you can use to envision your best later life. I've also used this process to create a clear vision for my own later life. I always try to practice what I preach–it lets me see if the things I'm proposing actually work in reality, and it also gives me the practical and moral authority to recommend it to you! I'll share my own process with you as an example.

Here are the three key steps of this process:

What are you solving for?
Where are you now?
What's the hope?

What are you solving for?

First, decide what core question you want your vision to answer. You can use my question, *"How can I become what comes after the butterfly?,"* if that resonates for you, or you can use a more traditionally logical question like, *"How can I create a purposeful later life?"* or *"How can I create a later life that satisfies me?"* Whenever I've done this kind of visioning, for myself or with others, I've found that having a what-am-I-solving-for question is extremely helpful; it provides a focus for your visioning, a clear challenge you're trying to address. I've found, in my work with clients around envisioning the future, that starting your question with "How can I...?" (or "How can we," when envisioning with a group) is a great framework for opening your mind up to what's possible, and that it balances aspiration with practicality.

So, reflect on what you're solving for, and note below a "challenge question" that will work for you:

My question is: How can I _____

_____

Where are you now?

The next step to envisioning your future life is to get clear about where you're starting from. We've done some of that already: the self-assessment I had you do at the end of Chapter 2 and the "fears" exercise I suggested at the end of the previous chapter. Now, though, I encourage you to take a step back and look at your whole life.

In order to focus this current-state reflection so it's not too overwhelming, let's look at only the things that are most relevant to the question you're trying to answer. Let's say you've decided to use the question, *"How can I create a purposeful later life?"* I encourage you to identify the aspects of your current life that will make it either easier or more difficult for you to create a purposeful life.

First, think about the positive things you have in your life right now—strengths, assets, attitudes, relationships, knowledge, capabilities—that could help you answer your question. Then, think about the negative things in your life—weaknesses, gaps, lacks, attitudes, difficulties—that might make it harder to find the answer to your question. For example, if you are very curious and like finding solutions, that could help you create a purposeful later life. If you have a hard time thinking about difficult realities, that could make it harder.

Here's what I came up with when I did this exercise, relative to my question, *"How can I become what comes after the butterfly?"*

Positive elements of my life that could help answer my question:	Negative elements of my life that could make it harder to answer my question
• I have a positive attitude about aging • My physical health is good • I have strong, loving relationships • We have sufficient financial resources • I'm curious and hopeful • I love to learn and do new things • I'm open to change • My work situation is extremely flexible	• I worry about losing my work identity • My physical strength/stamina is less than before • I'm impatient—with myself and others • I'm afraid of losing mental and/or physical capability • I worry about my husband's health • I worry about losing people close to me

Now, you try it - write down the positives and negatives you bring to addressing your question, either below or on the interactive PDF at thenewoldbook.com.

My question is _____

Positive elements of my life that could help answer my question:	Negative elements of my life that could make it harder to answer my question

I encourage you to be as honest as possible. Remember, no one needs to see this but you, and you want to give yourself an accurate starting point for your envisioning. I often talk about the concept of being a "fair witness," and I believe it's an especially important skill to develop when looking at yourself and your own later life.

The term "fair witness" comes from a book by Robert Heinlein, *Stranger in a Strange Land*.[3] In it, Heinlein creates a profession called Fair Witness. At one point, a character in the book, Jubal, is trying to explain the concept of fair witnessing to the book's protagonist, Michael. Michael is having a hard time understanding, so Jubal calls over a woman who is a Fair Witness, points to a distant house (they're standing outside), and asks, "What color is that house?" She replies, "It appears to be painted white on this side."

That's what Fair Witnesses do, in Heinlein's book: they are trained and then bound by law, when acting in their professional capacity, to speak only from their direct experience or from incontrovertible data. They can't indulge in speculation, cherry-pick the data, say what they hope is true, or avoid looking at what they don't want to be true. In other words, they're proscribed from doing all the things we generally do when thinking about ourselves.

Assessing your current state is a great place to start developing your fair witness skills. Too often, as we age (and this goes back to those fear reactions we were talking about in the last chapter) we either refuse to acknowledge how things are changing for us (*I'm really just the same as I was when I was 30*) or we sell ourselves short and think about ourselves much more negatively than is fair or accurate (*I'm really falling apart, and I'm nothing like I was when I was 30*). Learning to be as neutral, objective, and accurate as possible about yourself and your life gives you a much better starting point to move forward: it's hard to go anywhere if you don't know where you're starting from.

Once you've reflected on your own current state relative to your challenge, I encourage you to look at what's happening around you. Think first about your "supports"–those things around you (rather than within you) that could make it easier to answer your question: people, situations, cultural or political realities. Then, think about your "threats"–those things around you that could get in the way of you answering your question. Again, people, situations, cultural or political realities.

Here's how I answered:

Supports around me that could help answer my question:	Threats around me that could make it harder to answer my question
• My husband is enormously supportive of me having a great life	• Old people are seen as useless and weak by many

• My kids want the best for me • My business partners want to make my work transition smooth for everyone • Being part of a huge generation all confronting these questions provides support and examples • Many laws are set up to support older people (e.g., Social Security)	• There's still a lot of "ageism" at play in professional situations • The legal situation for older people in the US may be at risk (e.g., Social Security) • Our kids aren't nearby • The US healthcare system is kind of a mess

Now it's your turn–and again, it's best to be honest; you don't need to share this with anyone, and having an accurate starting point will be most helpful.

Supports around me that could help answer my question:	Threats around me that could make it harder to answer my question:

I've found that having a good, accurate sense of your current state relative to the question you're trying to answer is essential if you want your vision to be attainable. Once you know what you have going for and against you, you're much more likely to be able to create what I call a "reasonable aspiration"–a vision for your future that balances the freedom, hope and joy of aspiring with the solid practicality of what's reasonable, given your actual current situation.

What's the Hope?

Now comes the fun part; engaging that part of your brain that can envision the future. And just in case you're thinking to yourself, "Wait, I'm not a visionary, I never have been"–let me disagree with you. Every human being with a functional brain has the capacity to envision realities that haven't yet occurred. Every time you've imagined a vacation to a place you haven't yet gone, or a relationship that might blossom, or even a problem that hasn't happened but might. Every time, as a child, you thought about the bike you hoped to get for your birthday or the puppy your mom promised when you were old enough to take care of it.

We humans spend a lot of time inventing and then thinking about realities that don't yet exist! And it turns out this uniquely human capability of envisioning a hoped-for future in this way can significantly increase the likelihood of our achieving that future.[3] Here's a simple process for doing it in a more directed way to help you more clearly picture the later life you want to create for yourself.

Here's how it works:

1. **Select a timeframe**
2. **Imagine yourself there**
3. **Describe what you see and feel**
4. **Extract your key vision elements: who you want to be and what kind of later life you want to have**

1) Select a time frame: We are time-bound creatures, so it's easiest for us to envision how something will be different at a certain point in time or during a period of time. We tend to do it automatically when thinking of our own hopes and dreams (*When I finish this project... After the grandbaby's born... Next summer, when we're at the lake...*). By this point, having already thought through your own current state relative to your challenge question, you may have a good idea of the time in the future on which you'd like to focus your vision. You might pick a specific point, like "a year after I retire," or "when I'm 70," or a period of time, like "in my early 80s." When I did this exercise a few years ago, the timeframe I chose was "in my seventies."

2) **Imagine yourself there:** At this point, you'll get in a metaphorical time machine and get out on the date or during the period you've selected above, with the assumption that in this future time, you've materially addressed your challenge question. In other words, in this envisioned future, you have become what comes after the butterfly or created a purposeful later life. You are the person you want to be and have created the life you most want. It's important to let your imagination do its job and "put you" in this successful future. One way to do that is to speak to yourself about this future time in the present tense, and to note a few things that are true that time, to help "put you there." (For example, "My oldest grandchild is 21," or "The new decade has just started," or "It's been ten years since we sold the family house.")

3) **Describe what you see and feel:** When you have grounded yourself in this future time you've selected, notice first who you are. Notice things about yourself that demonstrate you have become what comes after the butterfly, or that you are the person who is living a purposeful life–what does that look, sound, and feel like? Write down your thoughts as they occur to you. Once you've noted the key elements of who you are in this future time, "look around you": What does your life consist of? How are you spending your time? What impacts are you having on those around you? Again, write down your thoughts as they occur to you. (You can also do it in reverse order, if that works best for you: think first about what your life is like, and then about who you are, living that life.)

4) Extract your key vision elements: Now you'll "boil down" your stream of consciousness brainstorm to pull out the key elements, those things that are most important to you in this envisioned future. First, review and select the 2-4 most essential (to you) elements that describe who you are in this optimal later life. Then, select the few things (1-3) that feel most important to you about how you're living your life–what you're doing, thinking, and accomplishing. (Again, you're welcome to do this in the reverse order–how you're living your life, and then who you are–if that's what works best for you.) These few sentences are the core of your answer to your challenge question: they summarize how you've become what comes after the butterfly, or how you've created a purposeful later life.

As an example, here's how I completed this exercise:

1. Select a timeframe

   In my seventies

2. Imagine yourself there

   I decided to "put myself" into the year I would turn 75. As "grounding events," I used, "My oldest granddaughter is 17, and we've been living mostly in Spain for 4 years."

3. Describe what you see and feel (in this envisioned future)

   About myself: I feel grateful and powerful, finding ways to move and be strong that work for me. I feel unhooked from time, and ageless–almost magical in my ability to experience the world and impact others in a positive way. I feel hopeful and open and vital. I am old in a way that I'm creating as I go and that's exciting and fresh for me. I can be unexpected, joyful. Age has ancient mysteries for me, and I'm finding new depths and new possibilities within.

About my life: So much time! I can go deep into things that intrigue me. I have the chance to find out and learn so much. I can be there for the people I love and help them discover new things, too. The world is waiting for me—so much to explore and discover. I can see and find new things, come to new conclusions, and share what I'm finding with anyone who's interested. I can keep helping others and working for a better world.

4. Extract your key vision elements

In my 70s, I am ELVEN—full of light, strong, deep and magical.

My 70s are about EXPLORATION—time to discover, support and enjoy the world, myself, and those I love.

Remember that your vision will be—should be—intensely personal. Mine may not resonate for you at all. In fact, it may seem completely unappealing to you: too woo-woo, too positive, not specific enough. No worries: it's simply an example. The only important thing is that it resonates deeply for me and provides a north star for me to plan and move toward so that I can create my best later life. And that's what I want you to create for yourself.

Before you try it, here are a few other examples of the key vision elements of other later-life folks I've spoken with, just to show you how widely diverse the outcomes of this exercise can be:

Me: I am kinder, slower and smarter than I used to be.
My life: My goal is to enjoy my life by helping others make progress. I'm a catalyst and precipitator.

Me: I've dropped down into a deeper version of who and what I am.
My life: I do what I love—I have the courage to find, honor and follow my bliss and to know that will best support those I care about.

Me: I keep evolving by asking "why?"
My life: I'm established as a "guru" with a supportive worldwide community; I love being seen as an elder with wisdom.

Me: I am a builder and participant in community–that's my joy
My life: I've figured out a great balance of a comfortable and comforting daily routine with new adventures, travel and learning

Me: I am grateful, sexual, less stuck in my patterns and more open to change.
My life: I'm enjoying life with my partner and finding interesting, useful, unique things to do daily.

OK, now it's your turn (as with all the other activities, this is also at thenewoldbook.com):

1. Select a time frame
2. Imagine yourself there (jot down a few "grounding events")
3. Describe what you see and feel About you: About your life/purpose:
4. Extract your key vision elements About you: About your life/purpose:

OK, So Now What?

Once you've decided on your "post-butterfly" or "purposeful later life" vision summary, I encourage you to live with it for a while and see whether it evolves. I initially made mine into a laminated card that I kept on my desk, and I tweaked it a bit after a few months and made an updated card. Now, it resonates with me even more deeply. I did my reflection internally, but if you're the kind of person whose thinking evolves better with interaction, you might want to share it with a couple of people you trust, to get their response and input.

Don't be afraid to let your vision evolve over time—remember, one thing we'll focus on later in the book is how to get good at change! Your vision should continue to represent your hopes and intentions and resonate with you as you move through your entire later life.

The goal of this part of our work together was for you to end up with a few simple, personal key phrases that resonate deeply for you and summarize who you intend to be and what you see as the purpose of your later life. It's your own *plan de vida,* your *ikigai.*

In the next chapter, we'll focus on how to make a simple plan to increase the likelihood that your vision becomes a reality, but before we do that, I want to reinforce the idea of "living with" your vision for a bit. Over the coming days and weeks, whenever you find yourself thinking about the years to come and what they will be like for you, or (especially) if you find yourself feeling untethered or anxious about the future, stop and say your vision sentences to yourself. Take a few minutes and let yourself see and feel how this envisioned future resonates for you: does imagining the "you" you've envisioned in this future life bring the feelings you want—happiness, joy, contentment, interest, satisfaction? If not, keep tweaking it, or even start over: I've found that only a vision that feels doable and emotionally appealing will draw you toward it and inspire you to make the effort required to get there.

Once you've created a vision that makes you think *Yes, this is who I want to be and the life I want to have*, that's a very powerful thing. We'll keep coming back to this central, simple vision of your later life as a touchstone for everything we'll be exploring in the chapters to come.

> **THE BIG IDEA: Creating a later-life vision that resonates deeply for you establishes you as the boss of your life in your own mind and provides a north star for all your efforts.**

---

[1] Buettner, D. (2010). The Blue Zones: The lessons for living longer from the people who've lived the longest. National Geographic; Illustrated edition.

[2] Berman, R. (2022). Having a sense of purpose may help you live longer, research shows. MedicalNewsToday. https://www.medicalnewstoday.com/articles/longevity-having-a-purpose-may-help-you-live-longer-healthier

[3] Heinlein, R. (1961). Stranger in a Strange Land. GP Putnam's Sons.

5. Make It Happen

"No one can avoid aging, but aging productively is something else." —Katharine Graham

By the time we're into the second half of our lives, all of us have accomplished lots of stuff. From the simplest things (making a grocery list, going to the store, getting what's on the list, taking the items home and putting them away) to the most complex: envisioning and creating a successful career; building happy and fulfilling intimate relationships; completing complex personal or professional projects requiring collaboration and revision.

In this chapter, we're going to be applying your well-developed skills of making stuff happen in the service of your later-life vision. There's a good deal of research these days showing that people who plan their later lives are happier, and tend to have better outcomes–both in terms of health and psychological and social well-being–than those who just let their lives drift.[1]

As we discussed in the previous chapter, I've been doing this kind of work for almost forty years with clients; both with groups of clients envisioning and then planning for the future of their enterprise and with individuals focused on their own professional future. And over the past ten or fifteen years, I've often used this process with clients planning their own retirement, as well.

I've noticed that when I do this process with individuals planning a retirement, the planning is usually much simpler and "looser" than when I'm doing it with organizations. That makes sense to me; an organization needs to be very clear about how it's going to allocate its resources and people toward achieving its vision and needs to have explicit, agreed-upon goals to measure whether it's moving in the right direction. Individuals envisioning the evolution of their professional lives need to be almost as specific: When will I have made this change or completed this requirement? What key relationships do I need to create or strengthen? What skills will I need to develop to be considered for promotion, and by when?

The planning we'll work on here for your later life will be less time-bound, specific, and goal-oriented. This is partly because it's a more confounded experiment: there are more variables, and there are (as we noted earlier) a lot more unknowns. But it's also because you're doing this primarily to satisfy yourself, and there are far fewer external constituencies to please or externally established milestones to reach (like a promotion or a yearly sales goal). Given all that, I've found that in helping people (myself included) plan for this latter part of life, it seems to work well to just sketch out some key intentions, with a few core steps to be taken to implement them, and then to let the plan evolve as you live it.

For example, I knew by the time I was 60 that I wanted to "cut back to full time" at work when I was about 65 (a little joke that makes most entrepreneurs laugh because it's true), and that I would probably want to work even less by the time I was 70. But it wasn't till I got closer to my 70th birthday that I started getting clearer on what that might look like. Also, our decision to move our main residence to Spain didn't start to evolve until shortly after I turned 70, and that has had a profound effect on our planning, one that I don't think I could have envisioned 10 years ago.

Now, let me add a caveat: You may be the kind of person who *likes* having specific tasks and milestones and is motivated by clear deadlines. In that case, party on. I did a personal vision and strategy session last year with someone who had decided to retire from her corporate job in her fifties, and she wanted to create a plan with clear strategies and measurable tactics, all with deadlines attached. She's done a bang-up job of executing her plan and is very happy with this initial version of her later life. (However, I suspect that if she does this process again a decade from now, she'll be much less specific and time-framed...but we'll see.) If you'd like directions for creating a more buttoned-up kind of strategic plan for yourself, I encourage you to read chapters 6 and 7 of *Being Strategic*, a previous book where I explain the more business-oriented version of this process.[2] There, I outline just how to create the kind of detailed plan that may be more your cup of tea.

So, for our purposes here, I'm going to outline the "looser" version of planning. But I want to start in a way that might seem very business-ish and anti-loose to you: by talking about strategy.

I've found that even in a loose version of planning, strategy is essential. Lots of people, though, seem allergic to that word, and even to the concept. In fact, when *Being Strategic* was published 15 years ago, Jack Covert, a good friend and the founder of Porchlight, an important retailer and arbiter of business books, said to me, "I was so disappointed to see you'd written a book about strategy–so cold and heady!–when your style is so warm and personal."

I responded, "Have you read the book, Jack?" He admitted somewhat sheepishly that he hadn't...and after he read it, he invited me to write an essay on their "ChangeThis" platform to help people see the idea of strategy differently. Jack has since passed away, but I learned a lot from him and was honored that I was able to change his mind about the relevance and universality of strategy.

You may (or may not) remember that I've already made an effort to sneakily introduce you to viewing the idea of strategy and being strategic in a more positive and useful light. In the first chapter, I shared something from *Being Strategic*: our definition for the phrase "being strategic." Let me remind you: We define being strategic as *consistently making the core directional efforts that will best move you toward your hoped-for future.*

Now that you've taken a first pass at clarifying your own "hoped-for future," I'll be helping you make a plan to achieve your vision by first figuring out the "core directional efforts" that will most likely move you in that direction. That's what strategies are: the core directional efforts that you intend to make so you can achieve your vision. And 'core directional effort' means exactly what it says: these are the few overarching efforts that are *core* to achieving your vision (you believe they are the efforts most likely to support your success) and are most *directionally* correct (you believe they will best move you toward your vision, rather than away from it).

You'll also notice that I said, "efforts you intend to make." Another way to think about strategies is that they are statements of intention. A good strategy should still make sense if you add "I intend to" or "We intend to" to the front of it.

Here's an example of a strategy I created to implement the "what's my life" part of my vision (which was, *My 70s are about EXPLORATION— time to discover, support and enjoy myself, the world and those I love*):

> **Strategy: Find engaging and challenging projects that involve lots of new learning and can be done at my own pace.**

This is a core directional choice I made, and it's also a statement of intention; I could have said, "*I intend to* find engaging and challenging projects that involve lots of new learning and can be done at my own pace." You'll notice that it's not a specific action. I'm not saying, "I'm going to build a chicken coop" or "I'm going to start a non-profit to support literacy." A strategy lays out a path, and the tactics are the bricks you decide to use to build that path. (Building a chicken coop or starting a non-profit might be tactics–"bricks"–I could decide to do to implement my strategy. They're not on my list, but they could be.)

Choosing Your Own Strategies

So, let's focus on your vision, and on creating a few strategies that will best ensure you move toward making it a reality. I suggest you start by looking at the "who I will be" part of your vision. Think about one or two aspects of who you are that you will most want and need to reinforce or develop to make your future vision of yourself a reality.

When I did this exercise for myself, I realized there were two areas I needed to focus on to make sure my "who I will be" vision (*in my 70s, I am ELVEN–full of light, strong, deep and magical*) would come to pass. The first had to do with "strong and deep." I wanted to make sure that I was making an effort to stay physically and emotionally strong in a sustainable way by doing regular physical activity that would keep me fit, nimble, grounded, and feeling powerful. I also wanted that activity to have a "deep" component–activities that wouldn't just exercise my body but things that would make me feel more vitality and even joy. The intention or strategy I came to that summarized this for me was:

Find ways of staying strong and vital that I love doing.

I then decided to focus on a second area as one of my strategies, or "core directional efforts," the idea of being "magical and full of light"– "elven," if you will. I wanted to make sure that I was continuing to be a person who brings clarity, hope and possibility into the world and in relationships; not to stop being a positive influence in my later life. My strategy for this area was:

Focus on being a practical point of light and hope in my words and actions.

I felt as though these two strategies were sufficient; if I could find tactics that allowed me to implement these two strategies, I would be creating a great momentum in the direction of who I want to be in my later life.

Then, I approached the "what my life will be" part of my vision in the same way and identified three areas of intention, which I also turned into strategies. To give you a complete example, here's my vision and the five strategies I created for achieving it:

Vision: In my 70s, I am ELVEN—full of light, deep, strong and magical

Strategies:

Find ways to stay strong and vital that I love doing.

Focus on being a practical point of light and hope in my words and actions.

Vision: My 70s are about EXPLORATION—time to discover, support and enjoy myself, the world, and those I love.

Strategies:

Create a "next act" with Proteus that serves my vision and the company's.

Fully immerse myself in learning the language and culture of my adoptive city of Oviedo, in Asturias, Spain.

Build even stronger mutually supportive relationships with those I love, especially my family.

TRY IT

Now I encourage you to do your own version of this in the space below or on the interactive PDF at thenewoldbook.com:

Write down your vision (it may have evolved even since you created it):

For the "who I will be" part of your vision, think about a few areas where you believe you'll need to focus your efforts to make sure this part of your vision comes to pass. Make notes below about what these areas are:

Now make simple statements of intention, or strategy, for these areas; 1 or 2 core directional efforts you'll make to move toward the "who I will be" part of your vision:

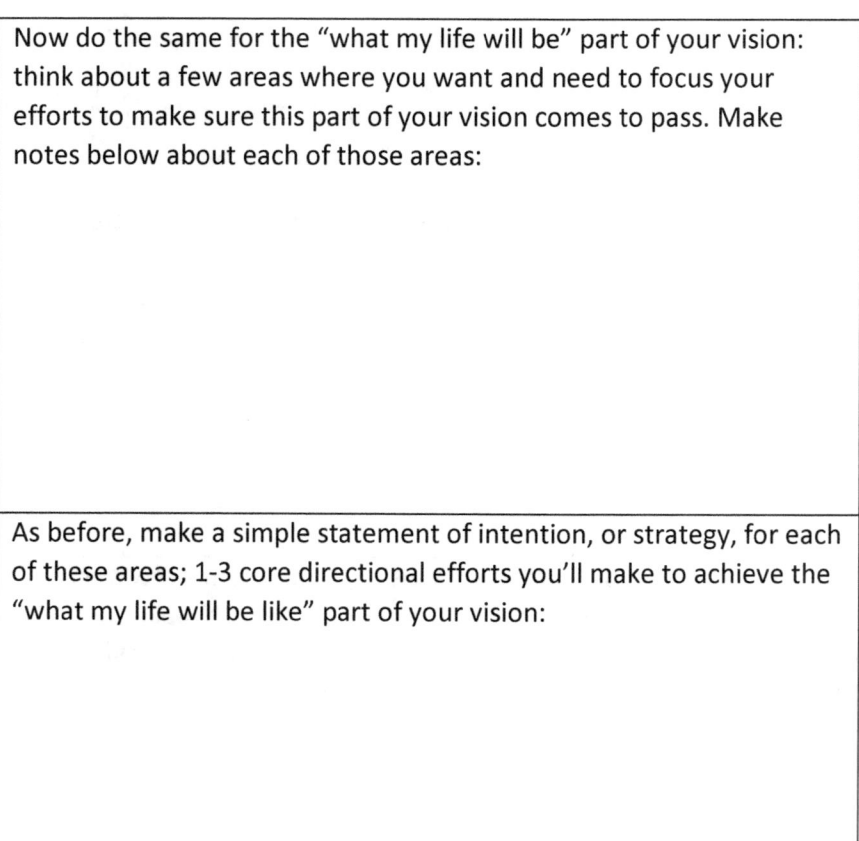

Now do the same for the "what my life will be" part of your vision: think about a few areas where you want and need to focus your efforts to make sure this part of your vision comes to pass. Make notes below about each of those areas:

As before, make a simple statement of intention, or strategy, for each of these areas; 1-3 core directional efforts you'll make to achieve the "what my life will be like" part of your vision:

When you've finished this activity, you'll have 3-5 statements of intention, or strategies, describing the core directional efforts you'll make to achieve your later-life vision. (NOTE: I've found 5 is a good maximum, and 3 or 4 may be even better–if you create too many strategies, it can seem overwhelming and/or you may be committing to too much.)

Will This Work?

Before we talk about how to use these strategies as a source of the specific actions you'll take, let's check to make sure you've covered your territory well. Sometimes, I've found that this first round of strategizing leaves a hole or two–you may still be missing a necessary core directional effort to have the greatest chance of success in achieving your vision.

When I did this activity recently with a friend, that's exactly what happened. Here's his vision and the three strategies he created to begin with:

At 75:

I am grateful, sexual, less stuck in my patterns and more open to change.

I'm enjoying life with my partner and finding interesting, useful, unique things to do regularly.

Strategies:

Find a way to restore and maintain the gratitude I once had.

Improve my initial negative response to change or difficulty.

Create personal projects that fulfill my vision criteria and can be done where I am.

Then I asked him, "Do you feel like these three strategies will fully move you toward your vision, or is there something missing?" After a few minutes' thinking, he said, "You know, there is something missing. To be as sexual as I want to be and to have the life I want to have, I need to be as healthy and strong as possible. My health isn't where I want it to be." So, he added a fourth strategy:

Restore my health.

Having added that, he looked at his vision and strategies and said, "Yeah, that feels good. It's all doable, and it will help me make sure all this stuff happens."

I suggest you take a few minutes and do the same thing: look at your vision and the strategies you've come up with. Is there a hole? Is some key part of your vision not covered by your strategies? If so, add it.

One final thought before we move on to tactics/actions. You're not trying to be exhaustive, and you're not trying to be perfect. You're just identifying three or four (five at most) "pathways" you'll walk down that you think will be most helpful to you in creating the later life you've envisioned. This is your best guess from where you are now. Six months from now, you may reflect on what you've come up with today, and say to yourself, *Wow, I completely missed thing X–Let me add that in.* or you might think, *Based on the past six months, I know thing Y isn't helpful at all, let me take it off the list.* The beauty of having a vision and a plan is that you have a hoped-for future and a set of core directional efforts to test out...and you can keep making it even better and more "yours" as you go.

Putting Bricks in the Path

You know how I said at the beginning of this chapter that when I do a process like this with organizations, it's much more structured and time-framed? Well, this part of the plan is where we're going to be most different from a standard business approach. When we design tactics–specific actions taken to implement strategies–with clients, those tactics always include what will happen, when it will happen, and who will be in charge. If it's complicated, we might define a number of interim "whens" along the way. We encourage groups to have no more than 3-5 tactics per strategy (but there can be sub-tactics) and to think about the resources it's going to take to complete them, so they're not over-committing. We usually have client groups create a PERT or GANT chart of all the tactics when they're done so they can see how everything fits together.

That's not how we're going to approach this. (Again, you can if you want to; in that case, Chapter 8 of *Being Strategic* will be your friend.)

Instead, we're going to use your strategies as thought-starters to come up with some initial actions that you think will work in terms of making practical steps toward your future. You don't have to worry about who will be in charge–you'll be in charge. You can give yourself timeframes if you want to, but you don't have to. You're just trying some things out. Once you decide an action is a "keeper"–that it really is moving you toward your hoped-for future, that you like doing it, and will keep doing it–you can nail it down more if you want.

Here's how this worked for me. When I reflected on my first strategy "Find ways to stay strong and vital that I love doing," I thought about how I like to exercise and be physically active, what makes sense in the two places I live now (upstate New York and the north of Spain), and what would feel best to me. My first list of actions to implement this strategy was:

In NY:

> Take nature walks
> Go to the gym in our apartment complex
> Go to yoga classes
> Hike in the woods
> Do dance classes

In Spain:

> Find and take a yoga class
> Join a gym if there's one nearby
> Walk to all my daily errands
> Walk for fun
> Hike in nature

Then I took things off the list that I knew I wouldn't do–either because I wouldn't really like them or because it would take too much effort to do them consistently. I also merged ideas that were very similar. Here's what the amended version of the list looked like:

In NY:

Take nature walks/ Hike in the woods - this is really only one thing, and it will work for me

Go to the gym in our complex

~~Go to yoga classes~~ too far away - I won't consistently drive 20 or 30 minutes both ways to do this. I could do online yoga classes, though

~~Do dance classes~~ - I don't think I'd like this

In Spain:

Find and take a yoga class - this would also be a cool way to meet people and improve my Spanish, I'll definitely do this

Join a gym, if there's one nearby - turns out there's a great gym a five-minute walk from the apartment

Walk to all my daily errands/ Walk for fun - these are really one thing, and I can/will do this daily

~~Hike in nature~~ - hard to do by myself, and my husband isn't up for this

So my final (starting) list was this:

In NY:

Take nature walks/hike in the woods

Go to the gym in our complex

Attend online yoga classes

In Spain:

Find and take a yoga class

Join the Supera gym

Walk for errands and fun

I felt reasonably certain that I would do these things, that I would enjoy them, and that they would move me toward being "strong and vital." Now, eighteen months in, they've gotten a little more quantified as commitments, and I am indeed doing them:

In NY:

Take nature walks/hike in the woods for 45-90 minutes, 2-3 x week

Go to the gym in our complex, 60 minutes 1-2 x week

Attend online yoga classes–90 minutes 1-2 x week

In Spain:

Find and take a yoga class–Tomas Zorza Ashtanga Yoga, 90 minutes, 2x week

Join the Supera gym - 90 minutes, 2x week

Walk for errands and fun - every day 3-8 kilometers

TRY IT

I'd love you to do a first pass at this. Start by looking at one of your strategies and brainstorming things you could do to fulfill it. Then go back over the list and remove things you're pretty sure you won't do, or that won't be very effective ways of implementing your strategy. You should end up with a doable starting list of 3-6 things to try.

My strategy (pick the one you created previously that you're most motivated to start with):

Things I might do to implement it:

(Make your list, then prune it to remove things you don't really want to do or don't think you actually can or will do.)

My final starting list of things I'll do to implement this strategy:

I encourage you to do this same activity for each of your strategies over the next week or so. (I've found it's a little overwhelming to try to "actionify" all your strategies at once).

Revisit your list every few months to keep tweaking it: remove items that aren't working, add any great new ideas you may have thought of, and note ways you've decided to quantify the things you're doing. I predict you'll be surprised at the impact this process has had on you.

Keeping This Top of Mind

One other way to keep this top of mind and help assure that you regularly engage with the process of making this happen is to create a laminated card with your vision and your strategies and put it someplace where you will regularly see it. If you're a more digital kind of person, you might want to make it the background on your computer or phone.

Let me offer a couple of other suggestions to make it more likely that you'll do this. First, you can use the principle of "habit-stacking." In his best-selling book *Atomic Habits*[3], James Clear talks about taking advantage of your brain's tendency to build neural pathways in areas of current behavior. If you link a new behavior to an existing behavior, that new behavior can take advantage of the strong neuron connections that already exist. So, for example, I've been able to link my new intended Spanish behavior of walking every day with my existing habit of doing errands (I'm strongly motivated to "get things off my list")–and since we've decided not to have a car in Spain, my new habit of walking gets leveraged into my old habit of getting stuff done.

Another way to increase the likelihood that you'll do the actions you've outlined is to tell someone else what you're planning and have a check-in meeting with them about how you're doing. A study by the Association for Talent Development found that people are 65% more likely to achieve their goals if they commit to them out loud to another person–and *95% more likely* if they have meetings with that person to review their progress.[4] Because we are tribal creatures and care about how others see us, most of us feel more responsibility to do something if we've told another person that we'll do it. It's important that the person you tell is someone who has your best interests at heart and will be supportive of you as you succeed.

Let me make one more plug for strategy as a useful (and not cold or heady) thing, before we move on: I would say that becoming more strategic, that is, learning to look at how to achieve important goals by stepping back and deciding on a few core strategies, has been a major key to my success in life. It has allowed me to get clear about what's important to me and then to let go of doing and thinking things that won't serve me. In difficult times, it has allowed me to ground myself in making a positive effort rather than in worrying and flailing around. I've also seen that my clarity about what I want to do and why has made it easier for others to see and support my efforts (in other words, it has made it more likely that they'll accept me as "the boss of my life." We'll talk about this more in the next chapter, too.)

I hope that playing with the idea of strategy in this context will be equally useful (and even fun) for you, and that it ends up being an important tool to add to your planning toolbox if you haven't used it previously.

> **THE BIG IDEA: Using your vision to create a plan that includes both strategies and tactics makes it much more likely that you'll achieve the later life that you most want.**

---

[1] Wu, J., & Chao, Q. (2024). How older adults fulfill their retirement plans relates to positive mental health: A path model analysis of social activity and self-esteem. *Current Psychology, 43*(7), 5963-5974. https://link.springer.com/article/10.1007/s12144-023-04735-6#:~:text=Retirement%20planning%20fulfillment%20promotes%20older,improving%20their%20positive%20mental%20health

[2] Andersen, E. (2009). Being strategic: Plan for success; Out-think your competitors; Stay ahead of change. St. Martin's Press

[3] Clear, J. 2018). Atomic habits.: An easy and proven way to build good habits and break bad ones. Avery

[4] Fogelberg, B. (2019). *Being held accountable for your goals.* Colorado State University Alumline. https://alumline.source.colostate.edu/being-held-accountable-for-your-goals/

6. Lead Your Crew

"Aging is out of your control. How you handle it, though, is in your hands." —Diane Von Furstenberg

Old people as either weak and dependent or crabby and rigid are such common day-to-day tropes in the Western world that we hardly notice them. Lately, my husband and I have been re-watching The Simpsons, undoubtedly a brilliant decades-long skewering of modern American society, but also–I'm noticing now that I'm old–deeply ageist. All the older characters are either mentally and physically incompetent (Homer's dad), difficult and demanding (Skinner's mom), or selfish and doctrinaire (Mr. Burns).

Sadly, the media only reflects common belief. The most recent World Values Survey by the World Health Organization found that more than half of the 83,304 people from 57 countries included in the survey had moderately to highly ageist attitudes: they saw older people as being less friendly, competent, and respected than younger people and–even more disturbing and important–as being a burden on society.[1]

This idea of later-life adults as being burdensome arises from an even deeper, older belief that seniors are in their "second childhood," that is, dependent and requiring care and direction[2]. This belief probably had more basis in fact in previous generations, when nearly everyone led much more physically active lives and there were far fewer ways to correct the physical problems of aging (from cataract surgery to hip replacement, statins to blood pressure medication). In centuries past, if you, as an older person, could no longer plow the fields, stir fifty pounds of hot laundry in a cauldron, or herd the cows, you probably *were* something of a burden to your family.

But even though we are now experiencing the new old (potentially many years of healthy life past sixty, with physical and mental capabilities intact) these stereotypes persist. For example, people are, without exception, surprised when I share with them the results of recent studies done on frailty in the US, showing that only between 6 and 14% of people over 65 qualify as "frail"–and only 24% of those between 90 and 94![3]

Why Am I Telling You This?

It's important to know that these stereotypes exist so that you can combat them effectively in your own life. It's especially important now that we're going to be discussing how to manage the group of people who will work to support you in your later life. In the last two chapters, you were just dealing with yourself and your own (possible) resistance to the idea that you can envision and create the later life you want. In this chapter, though, I'm going to encourage you to collaborate with other people to support your vision...and that interaction may, at times, run headlong into their resistance to your independence and/or direction: into their ageist attitudes. I don't want you to get blindsided.

Here's what I mean. As you know, the core principle of this first part of the book is "be the boss of your life." One characteristic of bosses is that they're responsible for leading other people to accomplish goals. As the boss of your life, you are responsible for leading those people whose skills, time and support you need to achieve your later-life vision. And there are many possibilities regarding who those people might be: service people, teachers, tradespeople, relatives, government functionaries, financial and legal professionals and–increasingly as we age–medical practitioners of various sorts.

Imagine all these people to whom you're looking for information, counsel, support, or results. Statistically, at least half of them will have some negative attitudes about aging and old people–specifically, the belief that old people are less competent and are a burden on society. Those people are more likely to enter into conversations and agreements with you assuming that they will have to boss *you*; direct you and even decide what's right for you. And perhaps (if they're bad bosses of you), they'll be prone to dismissing your concerns or ignoring your questions as they organize their part of your life, saying, in effect, "Don't worry your little old head about it."

Which leaves us with the question: How can you lead people who may not be open, initially, to being led by you...who may be assuming that you're not even capable of doing so?

Leading in Difficult Situations

Over the decades, I've often coached leaders who have found themselves in similarly difficult situations where their employees weren't accepting their leadership for one or a variety of reasons. Sometimes, the leader was much younger (or older) than those he or she was leading. Sometimes, the leader was from another organization or industry that wasn't respected or they lacked the particular skills or experience that the employees expected in their leader. Often, the problem was that the new leader was of another gender, race, or religion (a woman leading men, a black person leading white people, a Muslim leading Christians, etc.). We developed an approach to leading that worked well in all these situations, and I want to share it with you. It combines clarity with respect and collaboration around shared goals. Here are the main components:

1. **Get clear about the kind of people you want working with and for you**
2. **Sort for those qualities**
3. **Share your vision and your goals for the relationship**
4. **Agree on how you'll work together**

5. **Use the agreements as your foundation**
6. **Keep communication flowing (both ways)**

1. Get clear about the kind of people you want working with and for you

Often, as older people, we end up just accepting whoever shows up to support us. This is especially true when it comes to medical professionals. But we don't need to do that; if someone is rude or dismissive, seems incapable of providing the services you need, or doesn't collaborate well with others when needed, you can choose not to work with them. Making these kinds of difficult and awkward decisions is much easier if you already have a clear-ish set of criteria for those you'll invite into supporting you.

Think about the people you've most enjoyed working with–professionally or personally–over the years. What qualities did they share? Now, consider who you'll want supporting you as you age. Will you be looking for those same qualities, or are there some additional characteristics you might find important?

When I asked these questions of one of the people I interviewed for this book, an ex-CEO in his eighties, his response was, "The most important qualities I looked for in employees were competence, intelligence, and flexibility. Now that I'm older, those qualities are still important, but I find that I also want empathy and patience."

Another person I spoke with, a retired community leader in her seventies, noted another quality as having been most important for her in choosing her team members: great listening skills. She added, "Of course, I wanted people who could do the job–and who enjoyed doing the job–but I found it was even more important to find people who really listened well, especially when they were confronted with something new or something they disagreed with. Now, as an older person dealing with a variety of professionals–especially given that my husband has serious health issues–the ability of those who work with us to listen has become even more important. I also find that I want to deal with people who are confident but not cocky; who are secure in themselves as people and professionals, but who are still careful and recognize that they might make mistakes."

TRY IT

I encourage you to spend some time right now thinking about these questions for yourself. Feel free to note your initial thoughts below or at thenewoldbook.com.

> What qualities have you found most important in the people you've worked with over the years? (If your list below is extensive, you may want to review it and select the 3-4 most important to you.)
>
>
>
>
>
>
>
>
>
> Are there additional qualities you'll seek in those who support you now that you're older? (Again, if the list is long, you may want to review and "prune" it to the 2-3 qualities most essential to you.)

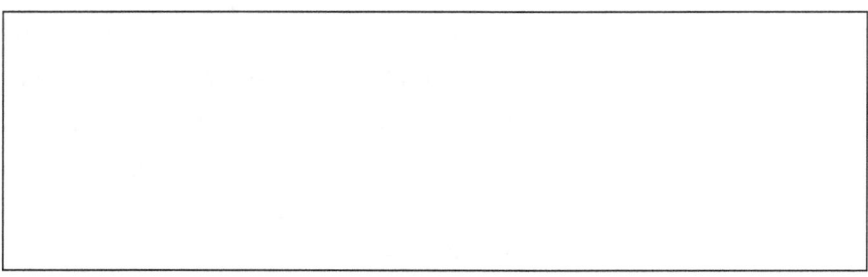

Consider this an initial list, a starting point for you to use in deciding who will be a part of your "later life" support system. I have no doubt you'll evolve it as you go; you'll probably find that some qualities you assumed would be important don't make that much difference, and you may discover some essential characteristics you've missed on this first go-round. But for now, let's figure out how to make use of this initial list.

2. Sort for those qualities

I suspect that at some point in your life, you've been in an interview–for a job, a school, a club. You know that good interviewers know what they're looking for and conduct the interview in a way that will reveal whether the interviewee has those qualities or qualifications.

I'm going to help you use your list to be that kind of an investigator of potential crew members: clear on what you want and able to determine whether the person you're talking to is a fit for the job. Don't worry. Our approach to this problem will be much more informal than a standard sit-down job interview, which is better for the actual situations in which you'll find yourself.

A Real-World Story

Last year, we decided to renovate the kitchen of the apartment we had recently bought in Spain. I asked our friend Antonio to recommend a kitchen designer, and I also started looking online for design firms. My list of qualities was clear: I wanted people who were highly collaborative, great listeners, curious, and extremely competent but also open and humble.

The person that Antonio recommended lost "points" right away by not responding to my emails and only wanting to communicate through Antonio. He came to measure the kitchen with Antonio when we were out of the country, and he then created a design that had little to do with the plan I had sketched out. Finally, he sent a proposal to Antonio (not to me, though I had sent an email asking for one) and asked for a start date, assuming that we would choose to work with him. I didn't have to ask him a single interview question to know that he was not collaborative or curious, that he was a poor listener (at least to me), and that he wasn't open or humble.

In contrast, when I went to meet with folks at a kitchen design firm here in Oviedo, the married couple who owned the franchise, Maite and Peter, sat down with us and spent over an hour listening to what we wanted, looking at our initial plans and asking us lots of questions, then showing us various options before finally asking us if we wanted them to create a proposal. Collaborative, great listeners, curious, competent, open, and humble. They ended up designing and installing our kitchen, and both the process and outcome were excellent. The few times we had misunderstandings or delays along the way, they were easy to resolve because Maite and Peter had those qualities we wanted in our crew.

So, rather than creating a list of interview questions, I suggest that when you're looking for a person or people to support you in some area, review your list of wanted qualities and write down how those qualities might show up in a person doing that kind of work with you.

Before I encourage you to do just that, let me share with you an example. Here's how I used my list of qualities when thinking about finding a cardiologist:

My wanted qualities: Collaborative, great listener, curious, competent, open, and humble

Type of support person: cardiologist

What to look for in interactions with this type of support person:

- Do they use "we" or "us" or only "me" and "I" when describing treatments or approaches?

- How do they talk about working with other members of the medical practice?

- Are they interested in knowing both my medical history and my thoughts about it?

- Do they ask questions to learn more about me and what I think, or only to get specific information (a checklist)?

- Are they open to me asking questions, or do they seem impatient or dismissive?

- If I bring up new research or approaches, do they know about them?

- Are they interested in discovering more if they don't know about them?

- If they recommend a test or procedure, do they tell me how it will work and what it will tell us?

In other words, before meeting with a potential crew member, spend a few minutes to think through how the qualities you're looking for would show up in your interactions with him or her. That way, when you're meeting with them, you'll be able to tell fairly quickly whether this person would be a good member of your support system.

TRY IT

Your wanted qualities:
The role of this support person:
What I'll look for in interactions with this type of support person:

A note: I think you'll find that your desired qualities are pretty universal for you. That is, that they will generally apply to most of the support people you'll be working with. We've found that a given person ends up wanting the same handful of personal characteristics whether they're looking for a physical therapist, a plumber, or a realtor. So, once you're clear on what those qualities are for you and you've thought through how they'll show up a few times, this part of building your crew will become much easier.

A caveat: Don't let perfect become the enemy of good when using this process. If you find someone who has, say, 3 or 4 of your five characteristics, they'll most likely be a good partner. This is especially true when dealing with a limited pool of "candidates." For example, if there are only two people in your immediate area who do the kind of home repair you need, choose the one who fulfills more of your criteria. (The rest of the steps I'm about to recommend will also help to increase the likelihood of a good partnership.)

Before we go on, though, we need to talk about the most difficult part of this initial sorting process–telling people you don't want to work with them.

The "No" Part of Sorting

Rejecting people is generally hard. It's why we so often do it badly. Breaking up with people via text. Never letting candidates know they didn't get a job, and just hoping they'll get the message. Bosses not firing employees who clearly need to be let go–sometimes for years. People who stay in bad marriages...or blow them up spectacularly, rather than mutually and amicably. I could go on.

And we, as older people, have an added layer of difficulty: often when we say we don't want to work with a professional after having met with them–especially medical, legal, or financial professionals–we get hit with the assumption that old codgers like us don't know what's best for us, and we should let younger, more competent people (i.e., them) tell us what to do. I've actually spoken to folks in their seventies and eighties, accomplished, intelligent people, who have had support people simply refuse to be fired. One youngish male lawyer said to a renowned artist in her seventies, after she had said that she no longer wanted to work with him, "I'm sure after you calm down and think about this, you'll realize that I'm only acting in your best interests." A shocking but all too common mixture of misogyny and ageism. She said, "I'm very calm and have thought about this a lot, and your response has only confirmed my decision," then stood up and walked out of his office. (Brava!)

Let me share the advice I've been giving people for many years about how to fire people well. You may argue that declining to work with someone you've just met is different than firing someone with whom you've already been working, and you're right—but I've found that the conversations (especially with professional pride and ageism thrown into the mix) can be almost equally difficult and require the same kind of approach. And sometimes, you will have to quite literally fire someone you've been working with for a while (like our artist friend in the preceding paragraph), so this approach will serve you in a variety of situations.

Prepare Carefully: Prepare yourself emotionally and mentally to ensure that everything that can go right will go right.

Perform Impeccably: Choose a time and place, and deliver your message in a way that creates the greatest chance that this ending will be as dignified and cause as little resistance and discomfort as possible.

Follow Up Properly: Make sure to think through and take any necessary next steps to minimize any negative impacts of the situation.

Prepare Carefully

Are you sure? Begin by making sure that you really don't want to work with this person. You may know rationally that this is the right thing to do, but unless you're sure, on a visceral gut level, that this is what's necessary...you will probably make a mess of it. Which is not to say that you have to feel good about it (it's an uncomfortable situation), just that you have to feel it's right for you.

Another thing to consider in this "are you sure" realm is whether you have an alternative if you decline to work with this person. If, for instance, they're the only person in your area who provides a particular service, or if there's one other person–but you haven't spoken to them yet, and so aren't sure who might be better. In other words, make sure you won't leave yourself without an option by saying "no thanks" to this person.

How do you feel? The next thing I suggest–and this may sound contradictory–is that you reflect on how you feel about, in effect, rejecting this person. Anxiety, guilt, or irritation are completely normal and understandable in this situation, even when you know it's the right course of action. Acknowledging and accepting any negative feelings you may have will make it easier for you to stay on track during the conversation.

What will you say? I suggest you take a bit of time to craft your message. It needs to be simple, clear, and definitive: a clear statement of intention, followed by a single sentence of "why." Omit any blameful or accusatory language: you're not trying to make the person see the error of their ways, or feel bad–you're simply making it clear that you don't choose to work with them. Here's an example of a good "thanks but no thanks" message:

> *"Thank you for meeting with me, Mr. X. I've decided that we wouldn't work well together. I'm looking for someone whose approach includes more focus on talking through possible solutions. Again, thank you for your time."*

What might go badly? Once you've decided what to say, sort through possible difficulties: ways in which the person might react badly to your message. How might you feel if they do react badly, and what will you do? For instance, what if he ignores you and just keeps talking as though you're still going to work together? What if she starts telling you that you don't know what's best for you? What if he says you won't be able to find anyone who will operate differently? Yikes.

Feeling and thinking your way through these situations beforehand and deciding how you would respond will help you not to be caught off guard, so you can continue to be calm and mature no matter what.

Perform impeccably

When and Where. When choosing how to deliver your message, your main focus should be on reducing the other person's discomfort. As much as possible, share your decision privately vs. publicly, and in person or by phone vs. electronically (that digital distance may make it easier on you, but, generally, it will feel less respectful to them).

Delivering the message. So, you're sitting in the room or are on the phone/video with the person. What now? The following approach will keep the conversation simple, focused, and brief:

- State your prepared message.
- If the person reacts calmly, thank them for their professionalism.
- If the person resists in any way, summarize their resistance without agreeing or disagreeing and repeat your message. (For example, "You think this is unwise and that I'll regret it. I know you may not agree with this, but it's what I've decided.")
- Then wish them goodbye and thank them for their time.

Finally, this is not the time for corrective feedback. You're telling them you don't want to work with them, not how they can improve so that you can work well together.

Follow Up Properly

Attend to Loose Ends. If the person you've just cut ties with is part of a larger group you're working with (a medical practice, for instance), do you need to let anyone else know you won't be working with them? If you found them on a website of similar providers, do you need to close the loop there?

On to the Next. Sometimes, it's such a relief to have had this difficult conversation that we can forget to connect with the next candidate. Again, if it's a medical or legal practice, be sure to tell the person/people in charge of setting up appointments that you'd like to have an introductory consult with another person in that same area. If it's someone you found online, go back to your sources.

Whew.

OK, you did it. Congratulations on being an honorable human being and doing a difficult thing to the best of your ability. Now you're free to find someone who will be a pleasure to work with in creating your best later life. Getting good at this particular task—letting people go well—will serve you for the rest of your time on earth.

3. Share your vision and your goals for the relationship

During the decades when I was working with and coaching leaders, I often noticed that the new leaders around whom people coalesced most quickly were those who shared their vision and their goals for the future of the company or department, and who then invited their employees to share their own perspectives and to talk through how they would work together to accomplish their shared goals.

Once you've found a person you want to work with in some capacity, I encourage you to use a simpler, more informal version of this same leadership approach. It's a powerful—yet relatively gentle and collaborative—way to communicate that you're the boss. It will subtly combat their ageism, if they're afflicted with that, and at the same time help you make sure your goals and theirs are aligned.

I experienced the benefits of this approach a few months ago. My husband and I had our first meeting with the general practice physician in the medical practice recommended by our insurance agent here in Spain (I had asked her to recommend people based on the qualities on our list, so we were fairly sure that he would be a good fit).

When we sat down in his office, he said *Dime*, (which means literally "tell me," in Spanish—but which is commonly used more broadly to mean "tell me what you're looking for," or "how can I help you?"); a good start. I began by sharing our overall vision for the relationship and then our three goals for the appointment. I said that now that we're officially residents of Spain (we had just gotten our long-term visa approved) and have insurance here, we want to get fully embedded into the city with essential services, especially with medical providers. So, given that, our goals were to get my husband established as a new patient, to get his three ongoing medications refilled, and to deal with some severe back pain he was experiencing that had been addressed in the past but had recurred.

The doctor responded exactly as I had hoped; as though we were "the bosses of our lives" and he was there to help us. He suggested that we address the immediate problems right then: wrote out prescriptions for us to fill for my husband's ongoing blood pressure and cholesterol medications; and worked with us to arrange a temporary steroid injection for his back. He then suggested that we return for a more in-depth intake appointment in a few weeks, especially if the pain persisted.

This doesn't have to be a complicated or time-consuming process. Patrick and I decided how to communicate our vision and goals on the 20-minute walk to the clinic; he had already figured out what he wanted to say about his vision and goals, and he told it to me so I could think through how to say it in Spanish. We finalized the message as we walked.

TRY IT

Next time you have an initial meeting with any support person, I encourage you to do the same thing. You might want to try it out below (or at thenewoldbook.com) just to get a feeling for it:

Person with whom you'll have the conversation:
Vision for the relationship (aligned with your overall "new old" vision):
Specific goals for the meeting:

You can use this same approach with people who you're already working with but with whom you may not initially have been clear about your overall expectations. In that case, you might want to start by giving a bit of context, for example, "I know we've already been working together for a while, but I'm not sure I ever shared out loud my overall hope for how our interaction would work, and for what we'll accomplish together. Is it OK if I do that now?" I've had this conversation many times and never had anyone say no. Asking their permission is especially respectful and a great way to begin.

4. Agree on how you'll work together

Once you've shared your vision and goals for the relationship, it's very natural to segue into agreeing about how you'll work together. Sometimes, that segue happens automatically, as it did with us and the doctor. If you need to prompt it a bit more, one good collaborative question is, "How do you see us working together to accomplish those goals?"

Two great things about this question: it gives you a chance to hear how your support person is thinking about approaching the challenge you've set for them, and it immediately communicates your desire to be collaborative vs. overly directive in your dealings together (this is especially important when you're dealing with people who may have unconscious resistance to seeing you as boss).

As they answer this question, listen very carefully. Note everything you agree with, and also note anything that may be missing from your point of view. If it's a complex topic (they're going to remodel your house or operate on your heart), you may want to take notes or record the conversation to make sure you remember everything.

Once they've finished, respond by 1) thanking them for their thoughtfulness and openness, 2) acknowledging everything they said that you agree with, 3) noting that you'd like to add a few things (assuming that there are things you want that they didn't say), and 4) sharing those things.

When you share your "adds," try to be as simple and clear as possible. Resist the tendency to be overly deferential or to minimize the importance of the items you want to add. That's a common way I've seen people try to deal with support people who resist their leadership–and it almost never works. It generally backfires: it communicates to the person that you don't really think you're the boss and that you don't expect to be taken seriously. Here are negative and positive examples of how to ask for specific items to be included in a working agreement:

Not helpful:

> *"There are some things I didn't hear that you said, and maybe I just missed it, but you know, sometimes it isn't entirely clear when something is happening that's not exactly as we expected, you know, when things don't go to plan And you know, one thing I'd like, if it's not a problem for you, it would be good if you could let me know, and I'd really appreciate knowing as soon as you can. I know you're busy and that you have other clients, but if we're not in touch about these things, well, it can be a problem, so if you could just contact me about problems when you get a chance, that would be great, and I would really appreciate it, you know?"*

As you can imagine, a rambling, provisional request like this is very likely to be dismissed–or not even really heard or understood in the first place. Here's a clearer, more succinct (and understandable) version.

Helpful:

> *"I noticed that you didn't mention how we'd communicate if there were problems. Let's agree that if you run into anything that we haven't already discussed, you'll text me as soon as possible. I'll respond as soon as I see it. And let's agree that you won't address the problem until we talk, unless it's an emergency. How does that work for you?"*

You might think that first one is an exaggeration, but I've definitely heard people say very similar things to their service providers and watched as those people disregarded the requests entirely.

Nail It Down

One final suggestion about working agreements. If the situation is complex, as I mentioned before, or if the person seems distracted or not very organized, it may be a good idea to write up your understanding of the agreement and email it to them. In the email, you can note that you're doing it just to make sure you're on the same page, which is true. It also sets you up for the ongoing steps of this lead-the-crew process.

5. Use the agreements as your foundation

Great bosses make clear agreements with their employees about what's expected, and then they keep coming back to them in a fair and consistent way to maintain momentum toward the vision and goals they've established. I encountered one of my favorite examples of this over twenty years ago in Jim Collins' book *Good to Great*.[4] He was talking about the CEO of a paper products company who had agreed with his senior staff that they would divest themselves of their paper mills–their manufacturing arm–and just focus on the consumer goods part of the business. It was a huge shift, but they decided to do it quickly: his team agreed to a six-month window.

Six weeks later, at another C-level meeting, the CEO asked how the effort was progressing. One executive said they hadn't begun and almost jokingly added, "But we have six months." The CEO looked at his calendar, smiled, and said, "Actually, we have 4 months, 2 weeks, and 3 days."

That's using your agreement as a foundation. Needless to say, they started working on it that day, and they got it done.

Now, since you're not the CEO (although you *are* the boss), your reference to your agreements isn't likely to get the same instant response, but it will usually help to get things back on track if they're wandering.

Pick Your Shots

You also need a good way to decide when to invoke the agreement. Some people tend to let things slide too long (the physical therapist has agreed to come at 10 am on Tuesdays, but almost never does; sometimes doesn't even show till Wednesday. But you haven't said anything because...), while others are too quick to correct or complain (standing by the door looking at your watch, tapping your foot, when the physical therapist shows up at 10:10).

When is it justified and helpful to remind support people about agreements they're not keeping? In these situations:

- When it's having a big negative impact on you - your time, your health, your ability to keep agreements with others
- When it has become a pattern - more than a couple of missed agreements over a short period of time
- When you've mentioned it before, and it still hasn't changed (this is a special case, which we'll talk about how to deal with)

The first two circumstances are pretty broad, and they will require a judgement call on your part–but they do provide some parameters and will help you be more patient and understanding if you tend to be too quick to react. And they will help you not fool yourself into thinking it's OK when it's not, if you're someone who tends to let problems go on too long.

So, what's the best way to remind somebody of an agreement they're not keeping? We've found that starting with some version of the following approach almost always works well: "I understood we had an agreement that _____. If that's your understanding as well, how can we ensure that happens?"

The reason it works, I think, is because, like almost everything I've suggested in this chapter, it reinforces that you're the boss, but in a respectful, humane and collaborative way. In other words, most likely to move things forward without activating or reinforcing the other person's possible ageism (or other biases).

Before we go on, let's talk about the third instance above. When you've already mentioned the lack of agreement-keeping (hopefully, you've used a neutral, considerate approach like the one I've just recommended) and the person still isn't doing what they've agreed to do.

What you need to do in this situation is ramp up the pressure while still staying collaborative, curious and hopeful. I've found that the best way to do that is to take the problem off your shoulders and, respectfully, lay it on theirs. Here's what that sounds like: "I'm confused, Mr./Ms.X. We had a conversation a few weeks ago where we agreed you would _____. I notice it's still not happening. I'd love to know what's going on and how you can change this."

The key phrase here is "how you can change this." We're assuming here that he or she initially agreed to the thing and agreed again in your last conversation. It's *their* responsibility to tell you how they'll keep this agreement that they've now made more than once, or to tell you why they can't, in which case you'll (hopefully) be able to find an alternative solution together.

And what if someone who is supposedly a member of your crew continues *not* to do what they've said they'll do, even after a conversation like this? If their lack of agreement-keeping is making it hard for you to create the life you want, I encourage you to use what I've shared with you earlier in this chapter: sort them off of your support system and find someone else who *will* support you.

6. Keep the communication flowing (both ways)

So, you've sorted for the kind of people you want and need and have made clear agreements about what you're trying to accomplish and how you'll work together to do it.

Great! But don't stop there. You now have the opportunity to build long-term, trusting, mutually beneficial relationships with them. This effort on your part will help to dissolve their ageism (if they're suffering from it) more than anything else. This is what good bosses do, and it generates openness, respect, and support.

So, how does that look? You listen to what they say with curiosity and interest. You thank them for their efforts and give them positive feedback when they keep their agreements–especially if they do something above and beyond the call of duty. You do things to support them when you can (write a great review online for your real estate agent, recommend your wonderful mechanic to your internist). If something they've done doesn't work for you, you give them honest feedback: here's what happened, here's why it didn't work, here's what I'd like instead. If they have feedback for you, you listen carefully, thank them, and work to integrate it if it's justified. Let humor be a bond between you (my husband Patrick said something that made my peluquero–my hair stylist–laugh the other day, and it took everything to a new and better level).

In other words, you use all the interpersonal skills you've built over your long and successful life to be a great boss and colleague and to help make sure the folks on your crew will be there for you when you need them. One resource you might find helpful is a book I wrote about how to manage people well, called *Growing Great Employees*; it has a chapter on how to listen well, a chapter on how to make clear agreements and give balanced feedback, and one about how to deal well with different kinds of people.[5]

Getting Better at Being the Boss

If you've already been a boss in other situations–in a paid job, in volunteer positions, or even as a parent–this may all seem like a good reminder and be fairly easy to implement in service of your later life vision. If you've never been a boss, and this is somewhat new to you, give yourself some grace. Let yourself try all this out, notice what works and what doesn't; if something seems useful but doesn't feel comfortable yet, try it out with a friend. If you have people in your life who have been good bosses, ask them to be your mentors.

Wrapping up this first principle...

Over the past three chapters, I've shared some new insights, approaches and skills to support you in being the boss of this part of your life. I've also offered a rationale as to why this–being your own "life boss"–is an important element of being able to create the later life you truly want. I hope you're leaving this section with a clearer sense of who you want to be as an older person, what you want this third act of your life to be like, how you're going to make that vision a reality, and how you're going to build and nurture the support system you need to help you achieve it.

In addition to the things we've discussed over these chapters, a big part of your success in being the boss of your life depends on your mindset about it. Which we haven't talked about yet but is coming up in the next section...

> **THE BIG IDEA: Once you're clear on your personal "new old" vision and have a plan to make it happen, it's critical to build and nurture a support system to help you get there.**

[1] Officer, A., Thiyagarajan, J. A., Schneiders, M. L., Nash, P., & De la Fuente-Núñez, V. (2020). Ageism, healthy life expectancy and population ageing: how are they related?. *International journal of environmental research and public health*, *17*(9), 3159. https://www.mdpi.com/1660-4601/17/9/3159

[2] Covey, H. C. (1993). A return to infancy: Old age and the second childhood in history. *The International Journal of Aging and Human Development*, *36*(2), 81-90. https://pubmed.ncbi.nlm.nih.gov/1297637/

[3] Watson, J. (Updated 2023, June 12). Frailty. UpToDate. https://www.uptodate.com/contents/frailty/print#:~:text=Although%20the%20prevalence%20of%20frailty,patients%20with%20cancer%20%20%5B6%5D.

[4] Collins, J. (2001). Good to great: Why some companies make the leap and others don't. HarperBusiness

[5] Andersen, E. (2006). Growing great employees: Turning ordinary people into extraordinary performers. Portfolio

Principle II:
Master Your Mindset

7. Learn to Manage Your Self-Talk

"When I wake up in the morning, I know that it's going to be the best day of my life. I never think about what I can't do." —Tao Porchon Lynch
(yoga master until her death at 101)

Years ago, I was doing an interview about one of my previous books, and the interviewer asked, "If you could only choose and use two skills, of all those you've learned and taught over the years—which would they be?" I thought it was a marvelous question, and I found myself answering without hesitation: "Listening, and managing my self-talk."

I would give the same answer even more definitively now that I'm older. Interestingly, both these powerful, fundamental skills are hugely under-recognized and underappreciated by most people. In the case of listening, we give it lip service: "Oh, yeah, I need to become a better listener." But we generally don't spend time actually doing it because we don't *really* think it's that important. (We'll talk more about listening in the coming chapters.)

For now, though, I want to explore the premise—and the skill—of managing your self-talk. For lots of people, perhaps for you, this is a new idea, so let me start by saying that we all talk to ourselves most of the time.

You know this, right? In most situations, a continual stream of thoughts in the form of words and images runs through our heads. I think of it as being kind of like that line of text that crawls across the bottom of the screen as you're watching the news. But inside our heads, rather than saying things like "TWELVE INJURED IN TRACTOR-TRAILER PILE-UP IN OHIO," our internal monologue is more along the lines of, *Wow it's hotter than I thought it would be today I wonder if I should have worn a lighter jacket did I tell Susan that we were going to my sister's house this weekend? Maybe I'll go to that Thai place for lunch today oh I can't forget to walk the dog...did I fix the leash?* And so on. If you're not yet aware of this near-constant interior commentary, I suggest you stop for a minute and just notice what you're saying to yourself right now.

OK. You might have observed that much of what you're thinking about is fairly neutral and day-to-day, like the example I gave above, but you might also notice that some of your internal monologue isn't so benign. Our self-talk can be negative, even downright self-sabotaging. For example, you might notice yourself thinking things like, *I'll never be able to do this, As you get older, life just gets less fun,* or even *Old age is awful.*

You may be wondering why this matters. After all, they're just thoughts, right? However, it turns out that, like lots of the aphorisms we learned as kids, "Sticks and stones may break my bones, but words will never hurt me," simply isn't true. You may recall that when I introduced this section of the book, Master Your Mindset, in Chapter 2, I referred to a landmark study by the Yale School of Public Health[1] that found that simply having a positive mindset about aging increased participants' life expectancy by 7.6 years. Since that study in the early 2000s, a number of other studies have reinforced the impact of mindset on both the quality and quantity of our lives. For example, a four-year study conducted with almost 14,000 older US adults asked study participants about their "aging satisfaction"; that is, their mindset about their own aging and about the process of getting old in general.[3] The study found that those in the highest vs. lowest quartile of aging satisfaction had a 43% reduced risk of dying from any cause over the four-year course of the study, as well as a lower incidence of having or developing health problems like diabetes, stroke, cancer, heart disease, lung disease, arthritis, physical functioning limitations, cognitive impairment, and chronic pain. Again and again, our mindset about aging has been found to have an enormous impact on how we age.

So, what's the connection between "mindset" and "self-talk"? One helpful definition of mindset is "a habitual or characteristic mental attitude that determines how you will interpret and respond to situations."[2] And the first place your "habitual or characteristic mental attitude" about a topic tends to reveal itself is in how you talk to yourself about that topic. In other words, when you think an opinion to yourself (*Old age is awful* or *It's all downhill from here*) it's because that's your current mindset—and it's pretty easy to see how that kind of attitude could have a powerful negative impact on "how you will interpret and respond to situations." For example, if you get the opportunity to try something new, something that could make you feel stronger or happier, and you believe that getting old is "all downhill," you'll be much less likely to pursue that possibility. You'll probably interpret it as wasted effort and respond by dismissing it.

Now for the good news

This all may sound grim, but fortunately, we have much more control over our mindset than we tend to think we do. We can alter our "habitual and characteristic mental attitude." Often, the most direct and powerful way to do that is to challenge how we talk to ourselves.

Here's how and why this works. It turns out that our mindset about lots of things—and especially our negative mindset—is often automatic and unexamined. For instance, we may believe that "old age is awful" simply because that's what we've been told by our parents or other authority figures, or what we've read in books or seen on TV. And, unfortunately, when that thought happens in our heads, we generally don't question it; we accept it as true (more about that in a minute).

Bringing those unhelpful, unsupportive thoughts to your conscious awareness, reflecting on them, and then deciding to shift them to be more accurate, neutral and supportive is a powerful capability. And it's especially powerful for us as older adults because having a more hopeful mindset about aging can, as we've seen, improve both the quality and the quantity of our lives.

I encouraged you just now to take a minute to listen to that voice. But 99% of the time, we're not conscious of our internal monologue: it's whispering away to us beneath our conscious awareness without us even recognizing that it's there. And because it's inside our head, murmuring along like subliminal advertising, we tend to believe what it says, even if it's not true. For example, if that voice in your head tells you *Nothing new or interesting happens to people over 70*, you'll probably believe it. And that means, as I noted previously, you'll be less likely to look for new or interesting things to do in your 70s, and you may even reject opportunities to do new and interesting things that come your way. In other words, your unexamined self-talk can become a self-fulfilling prophecy, so that your later life fulfills all your negative expectations.

So, how do we change the messages we're sending to ourselves and, in the process, evolve our mindset–about anything, but in this context, about aging–to become more supportive, hopeful, and healthy? Having been with me to this point, you probably won't be surprised to find that I'm about to offer you a simple model. Here are the steps involved:

MANAGING YOUR SELF-TALK

Recognize

Record

Rethink

Repeat

Recognize: The first step in managing your self-talk is to "hear" it. Most of the time, as I noted earlier, our little interior commentator runs and runs, and we're not even consciously aware that we're talking to ourselves, much less exactly what we're thinking. It's impossible to change this internal monologue until you're aware of it. So, you first have to become conscious of what you're saying to yourself.

For instance, let's say you're thinking about some difficulty you're experiencing (or anticipate experiencing) because you're getting older. You tune in to your internal monologue, and you might hear your mental voice saying, *I know I'm going to get much weaker as I age. That's how it goes.* Once you start attending to the voice in your head, you may be very surprised at what you're saying to yourself. That's what I meant earlier when I talked about aspects of our mindset being "automatic and unexamined." This first step is a process of getting your self-talk off automatic so that you can examine it.

Record: Writing down your self-talk, once you recognize what you're saying to yourself, is an important part of being able to change it, particularly if it's something you've said to yourself repeatedly over a long period. (I think you'll discover you have some of these unhelpful "mental tape loops," things you say to yourself over and over about the process of aging or the fact of being older.) Recording your self-talk creates a useful separation between you and that interior monologue. It functions kind of like cutting your hair: the hair that's cut off isn't part of you anymore, and you feel free to do what you want to with it. As soon as you see your thoughts written down, they feel less like an intrinsic part of you and more like something external that you can change.

Let's say you write down that self-talk statement above: *I know I'm going to get much weaker as I age. That's how it goes.* Having written it down, you can see it more objectively: a possibility rather than something you simply accept as reality. It's easier to see inaccuracy or illogic in the things you say to yourself once you see them in writing.

Quite often, when I've had someone record their negative self-talk about a topic, their initial response is some version of, "What? Yikes!" The first piece of negative self-talk I wrote down about aging, in my late 50s, was, *I've experienced all my 'firsts'—everything from here on is just going to be repeats.* My immediate reaction, once I had recognized it and written it down, was, "Holy crap—*that's* what I've been thinking? I don't want to say that to myself...I don't even believe it!" The moment I saw it in written form, outside my head, I was able to separate myself from it enough to start questioning its validity.

Once you recognize and record your self-talk, you'll also be better able to reflect on how this negative interior monologue is affecting you: perhaps you'll see the connection between your negative internal chatter and your abandonment of important goals, or how your negative self-talk has left you feeling cynical or hopeless about the possibility of architecting a satisfying post-career life.

Rethink: Once you've written down a piece of inaccurate, unsupportive self-talk and seen it more objectively, you can decide how to revise it to be more accurate and helpful. This step is the core of the managing-your-self-talk process, and there's an art to it. You want to create alternative self-talk that you'll *believe* and that will lead to a more appropriate and self-supportive response.

For instance, if you try to substitute self-talk that's falsely positive, like, *I'll get stronger every day as I age!*, you simply won't believe it, and therefore it will have no impact on you: you'll just revert to your original unsupportive self-talk. Instead, focus on what you could say to yourself that's both believable (by you) and that would create a more useful response. How about something like, *I may lose some strength as I age—but I believe I can find fun, doable ways to maintain maximum strength and vitality.* That seems realistic (and therefore believable), hopeful, and empowering.

Repeat: Like any habit, managing your self-talk requires repetition. Substituting more hopeful and accurate self-talk for your negative self-talk will be helpful the very first time you do it. *And* you'll need to consciously do it again the next time the voice in your head comes up with a similarly unhelpful statement. And again. This is an ongoing process for creating new habits of thought. Whenever you fall into an unhelpful self-talk pattern—either overly negative or unrealistically positive—consciously substitute your revised, more realistic, and accurate self-talk.

TRY IT

Because this is a skill and not just theory, I'd like you to give it a try, to see how it feels and how it works. Let's pick a piece of not-helpful self-talk you might have about aging and shift it from less supportive to more supportive. (As always, this activity is also at thenewold.book.com.)

Look at the fears you noted about aging in Chapter 3 (fear is usually a rich source of negative self-talk). Select a few negative things you're thinking relative to those fears:

Circle one piece of the self-talk you've written above that seems particularly unhelpful to you. (For instance, that saddens you, makes you feel powerless, or less motivated.)

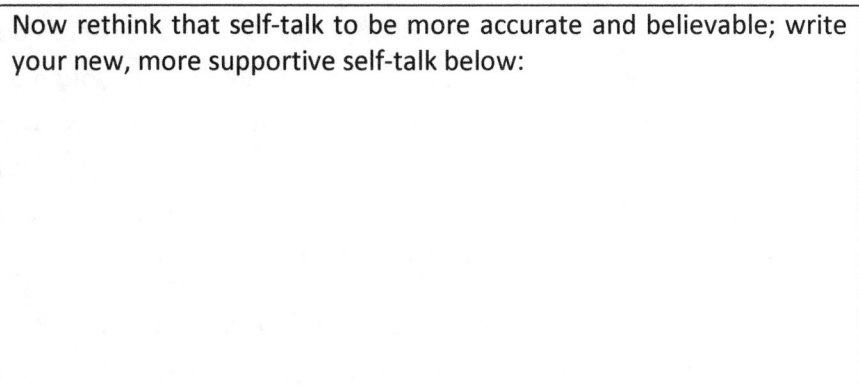

Now try saying your revised self-talk to yourself instead of the original self-talk. Do you believe it? If not, rethink it again to make it more believable yet still supportive. You'll know you're successful at managing your self-talk about a situation when you begin to respond to the situation more positively–that is, when you begin to feel better and to behave differently.

Making This Skill a Daily Habit

I've offered you a powerful tool in these past few pages. You may not even recognize the extent to which employing this tool can improve your later life (I'm going to keep reminding you about that Yale study and those added 7.6 years...)

So, there's having a tool, and then there's knowing how to use it, and–finally–there's actually taking advantage of it regularly. Let's talk about how to use this skill of managing your self-talk well and then how to make a habit of using it well so you can reap all the benefits.

Pick Your Shots

Just in case you were reading the previous section and thinking, Whoa, now I have to be aware of everything I say to myself all the time in order to have a better, longer life?, the short answer is: absolutely not.

As I noted before, most of our self-talk is pretty innocuous. There's no need to listen to it—just let your mind blather on and go about your day. So, how do you create the habit of recognizing and revising only your most unhelpful self-talk? Here's a secret that I've been using and teaching to people for over thirty years: *When you feel bad or act weird for no reason, notice what you're saying to yourself.*

That may sound too simple, but it's remarkably accurate and effective. I've found that when I'm feeling negative—hopeless, powerless, angry, sad, frustrated, demoralized, etc.—and I don't see any real cause for those feelings in my environment, that when I stop and listen to my self-talk, it is almost inevitably the source of those negative feelings. For example, one day last spring I noticed that I was feeling really anxious, and nothing seemed to warrant that feeling: it was a lovely day, I was hanging out with my husband, and we were talking about some stuff we needed to do before we left Spain to go back to the states the following month. No losses, no emergencies, no problems.

So, I took a moment and listened to my internal monologue and discovered that I was thinking *I bet when I go to the Policia Nacional to pick up my residency card, there will be a problem. They won't give it to me.* As soon as I realized what I was saying, I was able to revise it to, *It's unlikely there will be a problem; our lawyer has said this is the easiest step.* I immediately felt better, and I also decided to WhatsApp our lawyer, Belén, to do some "just in case" contingency planning. It was pretty much the only time that day I needed to be conscious of my self-talk.

You can also use odd, unwarranted behavior (as well as the kind of odd, unwarranted feelings I was just describing) as a prompt to listen to your self-talk. For instance, one of the folks I interviewed for this book (who is a big fan of managing her self-talk) told me that when one of her favorite friends, who she hadn't seen for a long time, reached out to find a time to get together, she noticed that she wasn't getting back to him.

She couldn't figure out why until she tuned in to her self-talk and realized she was saying to herself *Now that I'm retired, he'll think I'm boring; it will be uncomfortable.* She changed that to *He knows I'm retired, and I'm no more boring than I've ever been.* (She also has a great sense of humor about all this getting old stuff, which is extremely helpful.)

It worked. They got together and had a great time–and it turned out that he wanted to pick her brain about what it's like being retired.

Creating a New Habit

I've shared the process for managing your self-talk to shift your mindset, and I've offered a recommendation about how to select the most useful situations for using that process. But now we come to the real heart of the matter: how do you make this a habit?

There's been so much great stuff written about making new habits over the past decade. I encourage you to take advantage of those resources first. Let me refer you to two books that I think are remarkably helpful (and lots of people seem to agree with me; both are huge bestsellers). One is James Clear's *Atomic Habits*[3], which I mentioned in a previous chapter, and the other is BJ Fogg's *Tiny Habits*[4]. Both authors recommend focusing on small behavior changes, and both recommend making the new behavior as easy as possible to do. If you reflect on this chapter, you'll see that the behaviors I suggest for changing your self-talk are both small and easy.

Clear and Fogg also talk about the critical element of motivation. (Clear calls it "making the habit attractive.") In my own life and as an executive coach for over thirty years, I've experienced this as the key to any change you want to make in your life: you have to want to do it.

Aspiration

We call it aspiration, that motivation to learn or to do something differently or better. To do anything new, especially if it requires that you change your behavior, you need a fairly high level of aspiration. The confusing thing about this is that we often *say* we want to do things (learn the guitar, stop smoking, exercise more) but then don't do them. That's because just saying you want to do something doesn't mean you aspire to do it enough to make the required effort.

How, then, do you increase your level of aspiration, so that you have the motivation to learn and do a new thing–to build a new habit? In this particular situation (managing your self-talk), let's say you've been convinced, at least on a conceptual level, by my examples and statistics or by things you've heard and read previously. You now believe that if you talk to yourself more hopefully and accurately about aging, it will help you craft a better later life. But you're not sure you'll really be able to change your self-talk habits in this way.

How To Make Yourself Want Something

Here's what we've found works to increase your level of aspiration about something so that you can make a new habit of it:

- **Imagine the personal benefits to you of doing the thing;**
- **Envision a "possible world" where you're enjoying those benefits.**

These two elements are core to human motivation. Whenever we do something that demands effort–from walking to the corner store to buy milk to retiring in our dream location–we do it because we see clearly how it will benefit us, and we imagine the future where we're reaping those benefits. (*I only like to eat cereal with milk, and that new cereal will be delicious with milk on it.* OR *It will be fantastic living in Timbuktu; I'll be able to do the things I love every day.*)

You may have noticed that when we don't want to do something, we tend to think and talk about the *opposite* of benefits and rewards—we focus on the difficulties and obstacles to doing it, which further decreases our aspiration. Shifting our focus toward the potential benefits of doing a new thing and the positive future that could result, is a simple, powerful, feasible way of igniting your aspiration.

Let me give you an example from a dear friend of mine; let's call him Hector. In his fifties, my friend had the chance to cash out of a successful business he had helped build, and he decided to do that and to build the post-corporate life that would suit him best. I talked to him shortly after he had made the change, and he was deciding what he wanted his life to be like and who he wanted to be in that life (he's a big fan of our Vision and Strategy process and had already begun to apply it to creating his own best later life).

One thing he wanted to do was to get back into the study of piano. He had been a very talented player in his early life but had abandoned it because of a sexually abusive teacher who had had a powerful negative impact on him. So, for him to fully recommit to exploring and developing his talent was going to require serious work on increasing his aspiration.

Hector first thought about why he wanted to re-start his piano studies. He decided that three potential benefits felt most motivating to him: finding out just how far his talents could take him; having more music in his life on a day-to-day basis (music is very important to him); and showing himself that he had the power not to be permanently held back by his early negative experiences.

When we spoke about it, he said to me, "I know it will take daily effort—and that I'll need to find a great teacher who I like and can really trust. But the idea of putting myself back into the flow of music is very exciting and inspiring to me. And who knows what I'll be able to do? If I can get to the point where I feel skilled and confident enough to do a concert, even just for friends and colleagues, that will be wonderfully satisfying and empowering."

Imagining the benefits

Let's deconstruct what Hector did to help you build your ability to increase your aspiration—about managing your self-talk or anything else you might want to do. When faced with an opportunity to either return to his piano study or stay in his comfort zone of avoiding the whole topic, Hector focused first on how re-starting his studies would benefit him. The ideas of seeing how far he could go, of surrounding himself with music, and of overcoming past painful experiences were all very appealing—they really resonated for him.

I also noticed, in our conversations, that my friend was very clear about his own motivational system; not only in this situation, but in his life in general. I've noticed that this is true of people who are good at learning and doing new things. They tend to be consciously aware of what they like and don't like to do, which makes it easier for them to ramp up their aspiration when necessary. They can look for the potential benefits they know will motivate them in the endeavor they're thinking about.

One simple way to find out what motivates you, if you haven't thought about this before, is to look at something you are already making an effort to learn or do. It's almost certain that you see the benefits and rewards of knowing or doing this thing (since you're actually moving forward with it).

So, what are the benefits you're getting, or will get, from adding managing your self-talk in your life? Why might you be motivated to do it? I suggest you look at a few different things you've taken on recently so you can start to see the pattern of what motivates you.

Then, once you have a clearer understanding of the benefits that are most important to you in doing new things, you can look to see if these benefits might be available in managing your self-talk differently.

I've been talking to a friend over the past few years who knew that her self-talk about aging was very negative and unhelpful. She believed that changing her self-talk could improve both the quality and quantity of her life...and she also saw that when she said her anti-aging self-talk out loud, it was upsetting to her kids (it made them feel like she was talking herself into an early grave and having a terrible experience along the way). But she just couldn't get herself to make the effort to change. She had all kinds of excuses, many of them grounded in her negative self-talk about aging. My favorite (or least favorite, I guess) was when she said, "Maybe I'm just too old and set in my ways to change my self-talk about aging." (!)

So, a few months ago, I asked how it might benefit her to change her self-talk. She waved a hand dismissively at me and said, "I know, I know, longer life, less disease, Yale study, yadda-yadda."

I laughed and responded, "Clearly, those benefits aren't motivating to you." I leaned forward and looked her in the eye. "What's something you care about that would change if you managed your self-talk?"

She turned suddenly serious. "I hate that my bitching and negativity makes my kids feel sad about me and powerless to help. They don't deserve that. And, you know, I don't like seeing myself as a crotchety old lady."

"OK," I said, "So, if you could manage your self-talk to be more realistically hopeful, your kids might feel better about you and you'd feel better about yourself, too."

Nodding, she said, "Yes, I guess that's true. That would be good." She nodded again and paused, thinking. Then she said, "Hmmh."

I can't say she changed overnight, but I have noticed she seems happier and less burdened and that her kids seem less protective and concerned about her. She recently reported to me that she is now revising her most egregiously negative self-talk about aging once or twice a day.

TRY IT

Now, you'll have a chance to flex your own "aspiration muscles" in learning to manage your self-talk. Focus on what benefits you hope to achieve (or have already begun to achieve) from talking to yourself–especially about aging–in a more accurate and supportive way. Remember to select benefits that are personally meaningful to you; they don't have to be the "standard" benefits. This exercise may be relatively easy for you to do; since you've read this far and are doing this activity, you may already be recognizing the benefits of managing your self-talk on some level, although you may not have brought it to your conscious awareness. You can note your answers below or at thenewoldbook.com:

Personally meaningful benefits I hope to gain (or am already gaining) from better managing my self-talk about aging:

This is a very practical approach. You'll know that you've picked benefits that are motivating to you when you notice that they are motivating you–that you're making the effort to manage your self-talk.

But let's amp it up a little and improve your odds even more. Finding benefits that are personally meaningful to you is step one of increasing your motivation. The second step is letting your imagination show you the world in which you're reaping those benefits.

Envisioning a Possible World

When I was first talking with Hector, he not only identified three benefits he hoped to achieve by getting back into learning the piano, he also envisioned the future world where he'd be enjoying the benefits he envisioned. He talked about how much he would enjoy having more music in his day-to-day life and how fun and exciting it would be to prepare for and play a concert for friends and family.

That's the second part of this skill of "Aspiration"–envisioning a possible future where you're enjoying the benefits you've identified.

And you've already learned how to do this! It's the same "time machine" approach I shared with you in Chapter 4, Keep Envisioning Your Future. Once you've identified your personally motivating benefits, you can use this technique to imagine the future where you're enjoying those benefits: just put yourself in a time machine and get out a few months from now when you're reaping the benefits of managing your self-talk. What's happening? What does it look and feel like?

I encouraged my friend to do this part of the exercise, too. I said, "Imagine it's six months from now, and you're managing your self-talk. You and your kids are both feeling better about your attitude toward aging. How does that future look, day-to-day?"

She answered almost immediately, without even really having to think about it. "My time with my kids is more fun, and they're more likely to suggest new, interesting things to do–they're not worried I'll poo-poo them. And, you know, I feel more confident, more like I'm the kind of person who can and will do those new things. I feel more energized."

Exactly. I believe that having a 3D vision of what it would look and feel like to experience those benefits really ramped up her aspiration. As I noted in Chapter 4, we humans very often do this kind of future-visioning in an informal, almost unconscious way: by doing it more intentionally, and grounding it in benefits that are important to us, we can make it a powerful tool for building our aspiration–and therefore changing our habits and our results. (If you're interested in a more in-depth exploration of increasing your aspiration, you'll find it, along with other skills for becoming a better learner, in my book *Be Bad First*[5].)

TRY IT

Let's take this "envisioning" for a little test drive before we leave this topic. Review the personally meaningful benefits you identified for learning to manage your self-talk, and then:

Think about the future where you're enjoying the benefits of managing your self-talk. What does it look, feel, and sound like?

A Good Thing in Your Later Life Toolkit

Now you know how (and why) to manage your self-talk about aging and being older. You have some ideas about when to use that skill, and you have some support for making it a day-to-day habit. I hope that, over the coming months and years, you'll see the power of this tool and take full advantage of it in creating the life you most want.

In the next chapter, we'll be focusing on another tool for mastering your mindset—one that will build on what we've discussed here and take you even further down the path of useful mental mastery.

> **THE BIG IDEA: By learning to talk to yourself more supportively about getting old, you can increase your odds of living both better and longer.**

---

[1] Yale News. (2002). *Thinking positively about aging extends life more than exercise and not smoking.* https://news.yale.edu/2002/07/29/thinking-positively-about-aging-extends-life-more-exercise-and-not-smoking

[2] Vocabulary.com. (n.d.). *Mindset.* https://www.vocabulary.com/dictionary/mindset#:~:text=Definitions%20of%20mindset,to%20act%20in%20certain%20ways

[3] Clear, J. (2018). Atomic habits: An easy and proven way to build good habits and break bad ones. First Edition. Avery

[4] Fogg, BJ. (2019). Tiny habits: The tiny changes that change everything. Harvest

[5] Andersen, E. (2016). Be bad first: Get good at things fast to stay ready for the future. Routledge

8. Become More Present

"Anyone who keeps the ability to see beauty never grows old." —Franz Kafka

Most of us have had at least one experience in our lives of being completely absorbed into a moment as we're living it. It might have been a profound sexual experience, where you were only aware of yourself, your partner, and what was happening within and between you. Perhaps it was a moment of great beauty: a passage in a musical performance; a spectacular sunset; the dip and rise of a bird against the bluest of skies. In that moment, there was no past or future, no worry or hope; simply all your senses open to experiencing what was occurring right then.

When we recall a moment like that, we almost always remember it as evoking feelings of joy, awe, peace, hope, tranquility. Now, here's the truly fascinating thing: we might associate those positive feelings with the specific circumstance or activity, but it turns out that the simple act of *being present*, being fully absorbed in the current moment, is itself a deeply positive experience.[1]

This experience of being fully present in any given moment is called mindfulness. And though it's an ancient practice, long associated with Buddhism and other eastern religions, it has become much more well-known and popular in the Western world over the past four or five decades. As often happens when a practice gets translated into a new context, it becomes somewhat different. I'll be sharing with you the more "Western" version of mindfulness in this chapter, a focus on simply becoming more aware of the present moment in a non-judgmental way, without adding the more philosophical elements of the Buddhist approach. (If you're interested in learning about the Buddhist version of mindfulness, I recommend *The Miracle of Mindfulness*, a wonderful introduction by the Zen master Thich Nhat Hanh.[2]).

If the word "mindfulness" sounds too theoretical or overly complicated to you, you can consider this chapter to be about "being in the present," or "focused awareness." Use whatever word or phrase resonates for you. Recently, I asked my yoga teacher here in Spain how you'd say mindfulness in Spanish, and he responded, "atención plena," which means "deep, focused, attention." I like that, too.

But What Does This Have to Do With Me?

Let's back up a minute, though. What does mindfulness have to do with creating your best later life?

On the fact side, there's lots of evidence linking increased mindfulness to an improved psychological and emotional experience of being old, and to better health in old age. One large-scale Canadian study reviewed the aggregated results of seven investigations done exclusively with older adults, focused on the effectiveness of mindfulness training. The researchers found that "Results generally supported the use of MBSR (Mindfulness-based stress reduction) for chronic low back pain, chronic insomnia, improved sleep quality, enhanced positive affect, reduced symptoms of anxiety and depression, and improved memory and executive functioning."[3] Pretty impressive. And no prescription, surgery, or hospital stay required.

So, let's assume for a moment that what I've just said is true and that the data support the mental and physical benefits of practicing focused attention. However, there are even more reasons I'm including a whole chapter on mindfulness in this book.

I'm very fortunate to have been practicing mindfulness since I was a teenager. In the late sixties, in my hometown of Omaha, Nebraska, I heard about Transcendental Meditation, the first meditation approach to become widely popular in the US. Reading about it led me to reading about other forms of meditation, and my takeaway was that there was a positive experience to be had, perhaps even a life-changing experience, by focusing your attention on a particular physical or mental point as you let your thoughts flow by without getting stuck in them.

I started doing my own meditative practice, using my breath as a focal point, and almost immediately found myself feeling calmer, more centered, less easily upset. When I was 21, I learned a more structured form of concentration from a teacher named Prem Rawat, which I still practice and from which I continue to get daily benefit over fifty years later.

I've always found it helpful, in all the ways noted in the studies above, but most importantly, I find that practicing focused attention, or "atención plena," daily allows me to enjoy simply being alive, moment-to-moment, and to appreciate the gift of being alive without having to fill that life with a hundred activities. I find this is even more useful now that I'm older and am doing less, both by choice and by necessity.

Many of the people I interviewed for this book told me that the biggest adjustment for them in aging has been simply doing less. One of my interviewees told me that he's understood that he loves being active and will keep doing a lot as long as he's able–but I notice that even he has slowed down since the days when he was running a major media company.

Being mindful allows you to experience any given moment more three-dimensionally, so even if you aren't doing as much "stuff" as you did in the past, you can still experience your life as being rich and full–maybe even more so than before. Think of mindfulness as opening a door into each moment that you may not have known was there. By being more mindful, you may find that even habitual day-to-day activities, interactions, and experiences have a depth and complexity that surprises you. In addition to its other benefits, I've experienced mindfulness as an antidote to the boredom, loneliness, and impatience that can hinder us from having a great life at any age, but that can be especially problematic as we grow older.

What Gets in The Way of Being Present?

So, why don't we automatically experience this wonderful state of being fully in the present moment? It starts with our self-talk. When we were discussing our internal monologue in the previous chapter, you might remember that I noted that most of our day-to-day self-talk isn't extreme or negative: it's just a continual mental murmur that's often fairly benign. However, even the most innocuous self-talk has one negative aspect: it generally serves to distract us from the present moment. When I asked you to spend a few minutes listening to that voice in your head in the previous chapter, you may have noticed that most of the mental chatter you "heard" was about things in the past or the future or about made-up situations or worries that might not ever happen.

To reprise the self-talk example I offered: *Wow it's hotter than I thought it would be today I wonder if I should have worn a lighter jacket did I tell Susan that we were going to my sister's house this weekend? Maybe I'll go to that Thai place for lunch today oh I can't forget to walk the dog...did I fix the leash?* You might notice that the only present-focused statement in that whole stream is the opening one; "it's hot today," and even that one is framed relative to an earlier thought you had about how hot it would be!

So, even though it's often not negative per se, the problem with this kind of self-talk is that it pulls our focus away from what's happening right now and draws our attention into the past and the future. Now certainly, sometimes a past or future focus can be a good and useful thing, if it's purposeful: it might be enjoyable reminiscing about a much-enjoyed past trip to the beach, or essential to do some planning for an important upcoming task.

However, I'm talking about the kind of ruminating about past or future that's just chatter and is generally neither fun nor useful. It's just distracting. When our thinking pulls us out of the present moment, we don't get to experience the beauties and joys that are around us and inside of us right now.

And we're really accustomed to following those past and future thought tracks, even though they often don't serve us. An example: I spent 20 minutes or so one day trying to decide which of the objects in my bathroom vanity in New York I would need to throw away preparatory to our move, before I realized that I was missing the beauty of the park I was walking through right then, and that the decisions were going to be immediately obvious once I was standing in the bathroom, trash bag in hand.

Also, We're Jaded

The other element that gets in the way of our being attentive to the present moment as older people is our assumption that what we're currently doing on any given day can't be very interesting or engaging because we've already done it so many times. Once you've eaten thousands of omelets or taken thousands of showers, it's easy to just go on automatic when you're doing those things and to not really experience them at all. We assume there's nothing there that's worthy of our attention. And unfortunately, our western culture of consumerism and NEWNEWNEW supports this idea: we're told that the recurring, standard things we have and do day-to-day are boring and that the only way to have a great experience is to buy a new thing, go to a new place, have a new relationship.

The Good News

However, some things work in our favor as older adults when it comes to being more mindful, more present. First, research shows that we older adults tend to worry less than our younger counterparts. Partly, it's because we have less to worry about: our children are generally grown and our jobs, if we still have them, tend not to be of the 60-hour-a-week, high-stress variety. But it also turns out–for reasons that aren't yet fully understood–that when we do worry, it tends to produce a lower anxiety response than in younger people[4]. So, fortunately for us, our non-present thoughts, rather than jumping up and down and yelling at us, demanding our attention (metaphorically), tend to be tugging us gently away from the present–which can make them easier to ignore.

We also generally have more time and bandwidth available (given the aforementioned grown children and fewer hours at work) to actually practice mindfulness, so that we can develop the skill of being present and reap the benefits.

Finally, we can use our newly honed self-talk skills to disagree with any "been there, done that" self-talk we might be having. For instance, if you find yourself thinking, *I've walked in this park a hundred times. It's boring, I've seen it all,* you might revise that to something like, *I wonder what I may have missed walking in this park while I've been absorbed in my thoughts?*

Which reminds me, before we go on to exploring the skill of being mindful, I want to make a distinction between "focused thinking" and mindfulness. I was talking to my husband about this chapter recently, and he commented, "Oh yes, I get what you're talking about, I often just sit and think about a project I'm working on in a very focused way." That's a perfectly fine thing to do and can be a very enjoyable and useful way to spend time–but it's not what I'm talking about. Thinking about something is just that: thinking. It means creating and then attending to a stream of thought about a topic.

For example, if I were to say to you right now, "I want you to think about the most relaxing physical thing you've ever done," your mind would start to create images and commentary about situations you've been in that were relaxing, and even memories of how it felt and what you thought about it. But while you're attending to those thoughts, it's unlikely you'll be aware of your body in the present moment; you probably won't be experiencing whether or not you're relaxed right now, and if so, how that feels.

So, thinking about something means generating a stream of words and images in your mind. Mindfulness, or being present, means simply noticing the physical, emotional, or spiritual experiences you're having in a given moment.

Let's get started

I'll offer you three mindfulness activities here: think of them as beginner, intermediate, and advanced. If you've never before experimented with mindfulness practice, I'd encourage you to do them in that order, but if you're more experienced with this, you're welcome to do them in any order that appeals to you.

In all three activities, you're going to be closing the book and doing something that involves noticing your present experience (unlike the previous exercises throughout the book, where you've been simply thinking and writing about different topics). So, I'll share some instructions first, then encourage you to put the book aside and do the activity. Then, when you're done, you can come back to the book, and I'll offer a few questions for reflection.

All three activities involve these core elements of mindfulness:

- **Notice something that's happening right now**
- **Put aside any judgements about that thing**
- **Let any thoughts flow by you, while continuing to notice the thing**
- **If you get "caught" by a thought, simply return your attention to what you're noticing**

That's it. Being present is very simple, but that doesn't necessarily mean it's easy. Like learning any new skill, it requires effort. You may be shocked at first about the extent to which your attention wanders (that's what I mean about getting "caught" by a thought). Resist the temptation to get upset or to judge yourself–that's just another distraction! Notice that you are inattentive and then just bring your attention back to what you want to notice. Here we go...

Mindfulness Activity #1: A Physical Focus

To prepare for this activity, first choose a focus for your attention. I suggest you choose something simple that primarily involves just one of your senses. I also suggest that you choose something you find attractive and interesting. It could be something you'll look at: a flower in a vase; a picture on your wall. It might be something you'll listen to: a simple piece of music (a voice or one instrument); the sounds of nature if you're outside in the country. It could be something you'll feel: your breath moving in your body; how your hands feel resting in your lap.

Once you've chosen your focus, sit comfortably in a place where you can easily see, hear, or feel your focal point. Before you begin, notice any areas of discomfort or tension in your body, and change position or add pillows or back supports to make yourself as comfortable as possible so you can put all your attention on your focal point. Make sure that for the 5-10 minutes you'll be doing this exercise, you won't be distracted.

Turn off your phone or other devices; let anyone in the house know that you'd like to be left alone for the next few minutes; make sure there aren't competing noises within earshot.

You'll simply be noticing your chosen focal point. You're not meant to think about it, do anything with it, or decide anything relative to it. You're just noticing it. Let your noticing deepen as you see, hear, or feel whatever is there to be experienced.

Thoughts will come into your head; just let them go by, like clouds passing through the sky. As I said earlier, if you find yourself getting engaged in a thought stream, just notice that's happening and bring your attention back to your focal point.

TRY IT

Put this book aside and do the activity. Pick the book up again when you're done, in 5-10 minutes, and reflect on the following questions:

- Do you feel any differently than when you began? If so, how would you describe the differences?
- What did you find most challenging about doing this activity? What did you find yourself doing in response to that challenge or difficulty?
- What, if anything, surprised you about doing this?

You may have noticed in this first effort how often your mind wandered away from your focal point. Many people, when they begin exercising their "attention muscles," find it difficult to focus for more than a few seconds. I strongly encourage you to do two things: keep making the effort, and revise any self-talk that tells you there's something wrong with you or that this is a stupid, boring thing to do. Try neutral, supportive alternate self-talk like: *This is something I want to explore, and my lack of focus is perfectly normal.*

Even if you do have a hard time focusing, you may notice some immediate benefits. At the end of your 5-10 minutes, you may feel more relaxed and/or calm. You may have noticed tension in your body during the activity and been able to let go of it. You might find yourself appreciating aspects of your environment, or of the element you're focusing on, that you didn't notice before.

If you're intrigued and want to play with this some more, you can do this activity whenever you have to wait for something: in the doctor's office; waiting for your coffee to brew; on hold during a phone call. Get comfortable, pick a focal point, and attend.

Mindfulness Activity #2: A Moving Focus

Now, we're going to "up the ante," using the act of moving as your focal point. In mindfulness circles, this is often called walking meditation. It's a good thing to add to your repertoire because walking is such great exercise, and something you can do almost anywhere, anytime.

To prepare for this activity, make sure you're dressed comfortably–nothing that binds, pulls or pinches–and that you're wearing comfortable and supportive shoes. It's best to find a quiet, safe, attractive place to walk. Once you get good at this, you'll find you can be mindful even in a less-than-ideal environment, but let's start by making it easy on you. It's great to do this activity in a park, if one is available close by. If the weather isn't cooperating, you can also do this activity in an indoor mall. I suggest you try it at first by yourself or with someone with whom you don't need to talk (introducing a conversation at this point will almost certainly be one variable too many).

Your main focal point for this activity will be your body, and how it feels moving through space. Notice the movements of your limbs, how they balance each other, and how your muscles stretch and contract. Notice how your feet touch the ground; the order in which the different parts of your feet contact and then come away from it. Allow yourself to adjust your posture to make yourself more comfortable and your gait to be more free and relaxed.

You may just want to keep your attention on your body. However, if you find you can do both, you're welcome to expand your attention to your surroundings, noticing the sights, sounds, and smells around you. You're simply noticing how your body feels walking through your environment. You're not focusing on your thoughts about walking, or what you did before you started walking, or what you'll be doing after you finish. You're just observing and feeling yourself walking. As you walk, allow your attention to deepen: open yourself more and more fully to what it feels like to walk.

Thoughts will clamor for your attention; often they will be thoughts triggered by what you see or hear (or smell) around you (*Do I smell cinnamon rolls? I remember the cinnamon rolls grandma Lote used to make when we stayed at her house...*). Notice your thoughts and keep bringing your focus back to your body moving through space and–if you've incorporated this–into observing/experiencing your surroundings.

TRY IT

Put this book aside and do the activity. Pick the book up again when you're done, in 10-15 minutes, and reflect on the following questions:

- How did this feel similar to and different from other walks you've taken recently?
- What pulled your attention away from being in the moment, and what did you do about that?
- What new observations did you have about your body or your surroundings?

You may find yourself changing how you hold and move your body during this exercise; that's a common reaction. Because our focus is generally on our thoughts and not on our body while we're walking, we can get into habits of moving our bodies in ways that don't serve us. If you feel inclined to change how you walk during this exercise, I suggest you follow your body's instincts and notice the results. Your body could be trying to teach you better ways to move.

If you aren't able to walk unassisted, you can still do a version of this exercise. For instance, if you're in a wheelchair, pay attention to how it feels for your chair to move through space and notice your surroundings. You can also feel how the various parts of your body feel when in contact with your chair, how the sun or breeze feels on your body, and how it feels when your chair passes over an unevenness on the ground. The point is to be attentive to what's within and around you. I would encourage you to reflect on the same three questions above after the activity.

Mindfulness Activity #3: An Internal Focus

This is the most challenging of these activities because your focus here will be on your emotions, which are more closely tied to thoughts and, therefore, often more difficult to simply observe without getting pulled into thinking about them or trying to do something about them. The payoff can be tremendous, though: being mindful of your emotions can help you manage and move through them, rather than avoiding them or getting stuck in them.

Start by choosing a current situation in your life to which you are having a strong emotional response. It could be anything, from something small and daily (your partner regularly forgets to pick up the mail, even though they have promised to do so) to something big and scary (you know you want to sell the family home and downsize, but the combination of logistics and nostalgia just seems overwhelming). It's best to choose a situation that's at least partly within your control and one where having a less strong emotional response is appealing to you. (Once you get good at this, you can move on to things largely outside of your control, like national politics, or how your kids are raising your grandkids–but let's start with something less demanding.)

Sit in a comfortable, quiet place. Before you begin, notice any areas of discomfort or tension in your body, and change position or add pillows or back supports to make yourself as comfortable as you can so that–insofar as possible–you're not dealing with physical discomfort as well as emotional discomfort. Make sure that you won't be distracted by outside inputs for the 10-20 minutes you'll be doing this exercise. Turn off your phone and other devices; let anyone in the house know that you'd like to be undisturbed while you practice; make sure you don't have anything else scheduled during or right after the activity.

You'll be noticing the emotions that your chosen situation evokes in you. You aren't meant to be thinking about those emotions (i.e., why you have them, whether or not they're justified, what you'll do to make them go away, what you'll say to the person or people who may be–from your point of view–causing them, etc.). Just notice your feelings and the physical and psychological sensations they're evoking in you.

This may be a very new experience for you, and it may feel unusual, even weird. You may find it difficult to simply observe and experience your strong emotions without trying to change, avoid, or justify them. Your thoughts may be more insistent when doing this exercise than during the other two because our standard response to our emotions is generally thought-based: to think about them or to completely avoid thinking about them–neither of which is very helpful. For instance, you might find yourself thinking something like, *This is stupid, why am I doing this? Feeling my sadness, anger and confusion about selling the house is a waste of time.* Take a breath, acknowledge that internal monologue, and then return to simply noticing what you're feeling. It may help to tell yourself something that my son, a very wise man, once said to me: "Just move through that negative emotion because peace is on the other side."

TRY IT

Now, put the book aside and do the activity. Pick the book up again when you're done, in 10-20 minutes, and reflect on the following questions:

- What did you find most uncomfortable about doing this activity?
- How might this mindfulness approach to negative emotions be helpful to you?
- Have your emotions about this situation changed, and if so, how?

As I said, most people find this activity the most challenging of the three. The good news is that the rewards are correspondingly greater. The first time I tried this activity was almost 20 years ago, when my first marriage broke up. Because of how it happened, I was incredibly angry–and anger isn't an emotion with which I'm very familiar. I resisted feeling it, and that resistance was actually making me ill.

My son gave me the advice I noted earlier, about moving through my anger to find peace. I did a version of this activity several times over the following weeks, and even though it was both difficult and scary to feel how deeply angry I was about the situation, it worked. I did move through it (feeling truly angry wasn't deadly or even harmful, which was, I believe, what I had feared), and peace was indeed on the other side.

Making This a Habit

I hope you've experienced some initial benefits and are now curious to further explore this area of mindfulness practice. If so, let me refer you back to the part of the previous chapter where we talked about making it a habit to manage your self-talk. I encourage you to reread the advice I offered there in this context: think about the benefits you might gain from practicing mindfulness–benefits that feel personally resonant and motivating to you–and then think about the future in which you're reaping those benefits.

I'd also encourage you to connect the possible benefits and hoped-for future of having a mindfulness practice to the overall future you envisioned for your later life in Chapter 4. There are potential synergies there that could be very powerful. For example, you might recall that one of the interviewees I mentioned in that chapter had as part of his vision, "I'm kinder, slower, and smarter than in the past." He has incorporated a daily mindfulness practice of 15 minutes twice a day into his life as a tactic to support the "slower" part of his vision. He's seen that impatience has always gotten in way of his kindness–and even his full intelligence–and he's found that becoming more present has helped him to slow down and reflect on the impact of his actions, so that he can choose the best approach both for himself and for those around him, and therefore be both kinder and smarter.

I would also encourage you to follow the advice of BJ Fogg, author of *Tiny Habits*, to "bundle" new habits with existing habits as an easy way to incorporate them. For instance, if you already walk most days, build a 15-minute walking meditation into your daily walk. Or, if you regularly take some time to sit and read, start your reading period with a few minutes of focusing on your breath or a flower arrangement. Do you often take time to have a cup of coffee while looking out the window? When something is bugging you, add the habit of setting down your cup and noticing your emotions until you feel more balanced. (You may also find that you have a better path forward to resolve the situation.)

As you know, this section of the book is about how to master your mindset as a principle of crafting your best later life. I've chosen it as one of our core principles mainly because it's been shown to be so dramatically effective in supporting having a longer life and better quality of life (that Yale study, yet again...). But I've also chosen it because it's something over which we have almost complete control. As we age, we will almost certainly have more health issues, even if we are basically healthy, and our physical abilities may be compromised in a variety of ways. But for most of us, our minds remain strong and active, and we can learn to use our awareness and our thoughts to best serve us. In fact, mastering our mindset in these ways can also help ensure that our mental facilities *stay* strong and agile and that we continue to experience the subtlety and richness hiding in the day-to-day.

I want to share with you one more wonderful example of the power of mindfulness to make our later lives more joyful and full of meaning. Pablo Casals, who was considered the world's premiere cellist for many decades, was interviewed shortly before his death in 1973 at the age of 96. The interviewer asked him if he was tired or bored of playing the Bach cello suites, which were a core part of his repertoire and which he had played hundreds of times. Surprised, Casals replied, "But I have never played the same piece of music twice. Always new."

That's mindfulness.

In the next chapter, we'll talk about the third tool in our "mindset mastery" toolkit–something that may be the most powerful of all.

THE BIG IDEA: The ancient practice of mindfulness, brought into the 21st century, can support your physical and mental health–while providing a profoundly nourishing experience of joy.

[1] Lindsay, E. K., Chin, B., Greco, C. M., Young, S., Brown, K. W., Wright, A. G., ... & Creswell, J. D. (2018). How mindfulness training promotes positive emotions: Dismantling acceptance skills training in two randomized controlled trials. *Journal of personality and social psychology*, *115*(6), 944. https://pubmed.ncbi.nlm.nih.gov/30550321/

[2] Hanh, T. N., (1999). The miracle of mindfulness: An introduction of the practice of meditation. Beacon Press; First Edition 1987

[3] Hazlett-Stevens, H., Singer, J., & Chong, A. (2019). Mindfulness-based stress reduction and mindfulness-based cognitive therapy with older adults: a qualitative review of randomized controlled outcome research. *Clinical gerontologist*, *42*(4), 347-358. https://www.tandfonline.com/doi/full/10.1080/07317115.2018.1518282?src=recsys

[4] Gould, C. E., Gerolimatos, L. A., & Edelstein, B. A. (2015). Experimental examination of worry among older and young adults. *International Psychogeriatrics*, *27*(7), 1177-1190. https://www.cambridge.org/core/journals/international-psychogeriatrics/article/abs/experimental-examination-of-worry-among-older-and-young-adults/5F78C8C60DE2D28E102895CAAF41EBC1

9. Cultivate Gratitude

"The longer I live, the more beautiful life becomes."
—Frank Lloyd Wright

My much-loved older brother, David, died in the summer of 2021. He had been living with severe rheumatoid arthritis for many years, which he was relentless in addressing both physically and mentally, and then in early 2020 was diagnosed with advanced cancer in his bones, brain and liver. He was able, with tremendous focus and great medical care, to drive it into remission by the beginning of the following year–but his body, already weakened by the years of RA, was too compromised by the chemotherapy (which David called "life-saving poison") to be able to recover. He got gradually weaker and weaker, and finally, in the beginning of June, came home from the hospital, where he died peacefully a few weeks later, surrounded by his long-time partner, his children, his siblings, and his dearest friends.

I miss him still, and I'm sure I'll miss him for the rest of my life. The thing I most admire about him, and find most remarkable, was that until the very last day of his life, even with all the painful and difficult health challenges he was experiencing, David was unendingly grateful. He was grateful for his loved ones; for all the relationships and experiences he had had throughout his life; for the daily small joys of great music, delicious food, wonderful conversation; for the experience of meditation with which he had been gifted by his spiritual master; for the central, astonishing fact of simply being alive.

The Mystery of Gratitude

How can that be? That one person, living with a variety of challenges, even facing death, can still reflect on their life and feel gratitude? While another person whose life seems filled with privilege, advantage, and benefit feels victimized, dissatisfied, unfaired-against...not grateful?

The dictionary defines gratitude as "the quality of being thankful." Gratitude is having the experience of "I feel so fortunate that..." or "I so much appreciate that..." Why, then, do some people consistently have that experience and others much less so, seemingly almost independent of their circumstances...and why does it matter? More specifically, why does it matter to us in the later part of our lives?

As scientists have focused in recent years on the benefits of gratitude, more studies have also been done on the obstacles to feeling gratitude; the reasons why it's more difficult for some people than others. It turns out that there may be physiological and psychological barriers that make it harder for certain people to experience gratitude. There are specific genetic and brain structure components that seem to predispose people toward or away from gratitude, and it also seems to be the case that some personality traits are associated with lower levels of gratitude–specifically materialism, envy, and narcissism.[1]

However, research also shows that we can overcome all these impediments, both physiological and psychological, by strengthening our mental and emotional "gratitude muscles," which will be the focus of this chapter. But first: why bother?

The Benefits of Being Grateful

An article from the Harvard Medical School that I mentioned in Chapter 2 references a variety of studies that reinforce the physical, mental and emotional benefits of feeling gratitude. And these benefits, researchers have found, are even more profound for seniors.[2] In study after study, older people who practice being grateful derive similar key benefits from that practice: better and more restful sleep; improved overall physical health; stronger and more positive connections with others; more psychological resilience in the face of difficulty; and sustainable increases in happiness.[3, 4]

Here's an excerpt from that Harvard Medical School article that provides a very simple but profound example of the power of just a small focus on gratitude:

"Two psychologists, Dr. Robert A. Emmons of the University of California Davis, and Dr. Michael E. McCullough of the University of Miami, have done much of the research on gratitude. In one study, they asked all participants to write a few sentences each week, focusing on particular topics.

One group wrote about things they were grateful for that had occurred during the week. A second group wrote about daily irritations or things that had displeased them, and the third group wrote about events that had affected them (with no emphasis on them being positive or negative). After 10 weeks, those who wrote about gratitude were more optimistic and felt better about their lives. Surprisingly, they also exercised more and had fewer visits to physicians than those who focused on sources of aggravation.[2]"

Many of my interviewees for this book have shared with me their own experiences that reflect these findings. One man, a world-renowned consultant in his eighties, noted that he and his wife make a daily habit of noting the things they're grateful for—and he told me that this has been particularly helpful as he's gradually lost his sight over the past few years. He's focusing more on what he can still do and even acknowledging the positive elements that his near-blindness brings into his life. One example: many of his former graduate students and colleagues have offered to read to him, and he's grateful for the renewed connections and the "marvelous conversations" that brings.

Another interviewee, a former executive, says she feels grateful to have the time and resources to pursue her artistic side–and grateful that it connects her with the memory of her beloved dad, a lawyer who was also a gifted artist.

When I ask people what it feels like to them to experience gratitude, especially as older adults, the words I hear over and over are "contented," "joyful," "peaceful," and "connected." This reflects a phenomenon Brené Brown noted: "It's not joy that makes us grateful, it's gratitude that makes us joyful." This is a critical understanding, and it goes back to what I noticed about my brother David. Many people think that their lives have to be ideal, or nearly so, for them to feel grateful, but the lovely secret of gratitude is that we can experience it even when we're dealing with painful, complex challenges in our lives. Simply feeling gratitude in the midst of difficult circumstances brings us joy.

Getting Grateful

So, let's build your gratitude capability. Let me start by reiterating that this is possible for anyone. Since gratitude is such a powerful component of crafting a great later life, it's good to know that even those of us who are physiologically or psychologically "gratitude-challenged" can build our ability to feel gratitude. In other words, if you recognize that feeling gratitude isn't something that comes naturally to you, this next part will be especially helpful.

More good news: everything we've talked about and learned in the last two chapters will come in handy now. Being able to manage your self-talk and being able to be present in a given moment are the foundational skills key to establishing a daily gratitude practice. We'll also use what you've learned about increasing your aspiration (to help motivate you to create a gratitude habit if you don't already have one), and we'll leverage the experience you've gained in making habits over the past few chapters.

Aspiration—wanting to feel grateful

Let's start by noticing your current level of aspiration. Are you already regularly taking time to be grateful, to acknowledge ways in which you feel fortunate? Simply notice your current behavior in this area; no need to judge. We're just trying to figure out where you're starting from.

If you realize that you're already practicing gratitude fairly regularly, you can skip this part if you'd like and go right to the next section on managing your self-talk toward gratitude. However, if you see that feeling gratitude is something you rarely do, let's start by focusing on building your "wanting to."

You may remember that when I introduced the idea of "aspiration"—of getting yourself to want to do something—in Chapter 7, I encouraged you to figure out some benefits of doing that thing that would be personally motivating to you, and then to envision a future where you were reaping those benefits. So, let's do that relative to gratitude: let's first find some benefits that are personally motivating to you.

Start by reflecting on everything I've noted to this point about the benefits of gratitude. You may have read other articles or books about the benefits of gratitude, as well. You might also think about a person or people in your life who seem grateful.

I suggest you also reflect on the vision for your future that you established in Chapter 4. Ask yourself: Will experiencing gratitude more regularly have the benefit of helping me achieve that vision? For example, you might remember that one of the folks I talked to defined part of his vision as, "I'm enjoying life with my partner and finding interesting, useful, unique things to do daily." He realized that creating a regular gratitude practice was key to him fully enjoying life with his partner—a benefit that was definitely personally motivating for him.

TRY IT

As you reflect on all you've read, heard, thought, or observed about the benefits of feeling grateful, which ones are most interesting or meaningful to you? You might notice yourself thinking something like, "Yeah, I'd definitely like to feel more X," or "It would be wonderful if gratitude would support me to be more Y." Those Xs and Ys are likely to be benefits that resonate for you.

Again, don't judge your own motivations. I talked to one man who told me that his initial motivation for making the effort to feel more grateful was that he felt envious of his wife, whose gratitude practice seemed to be making her less affected by difficult circumstances–and he wanted to have that same experience! It worked just fine for him as an initial motivator.

You can note your answers below or at thenewoldbook.com:

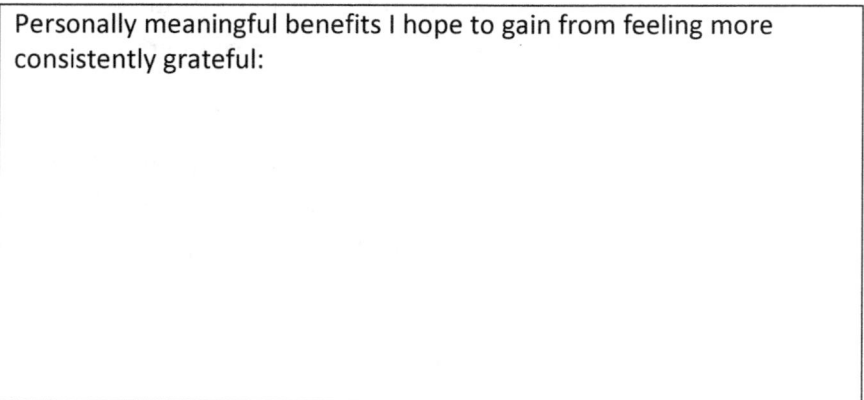

Personally meaningful benefits I hope to gain from feeling more consistently grateful:

Now, spend a little time, in effect, future-dreaming. What will it look, feel and sound like when you're practicing gratitude regularly and getting the benefits you're hoping for? When my interviewee who wanted to practice gratitude to be better able to enjoy life with his partner did this second part of the exercise, he envisioned "less time spent bitching about the indignities of being old, and more time noticing what a wonderful companion my partner is and how much fun it is to be together."

Imagine the improved future you'll have as a result of your gratitude practice, and note below what you envision:

```
The future where I'm reaping the benefits of practicing gratitude:




```

Remember, when you're working to increase your aspiration, the proof is in the pudding. If you find, over the next few weeks, that reflecting on these benefits and the future they might yield doesn't motivate you to make a gratitude practice...then you've chosen benefits that aren't really meaningful to you. Think about it again, surface other possible benefits, and try focusing on them. And I'll say it once more: don't just think about the benefits that you believe "should" be motivating to you. Your most effective benefits may seem selfish (think about my interviewee who envied his wife) or just plain odd (I started exercising twenty years ago because I realized I could read while on the elliptical trainer). The point of this activity is to simply find what will work for you.

Managing Your Negative Self-Talk Toward Gratitude

It probably won't surprise you to find out that the experience of gratitude (or the lack thereof) starts in how we talk to ourselves about our life and our circumstances. Going back to the example of my brother David, and his gift of gratitude; a number of years ago I was talking to him about his RA (rheumatoid arthritis), and he said, "Probably the most difficult thing about this has been that I can't really play the guitar any longer." Then he added, "But I choose to focus on the support I've gotten from so many wonderful people, therapists and medical professionals, that has allowed me to continue to do other things that are important to me, like tuning pianos and teaching piano technicians." (His profession, at which he was uniquely gifted.)

David was letting me know that instead of only talking to himself about what he had lost and what saddened him regarding his RA, he *chose* to also remind himself to be grateful for the things he could still do and the support of others that allowed that.

He was managing his self-talk in very much the same way we discussed it in Chapter 7. He noticed how he was talking to himself, and he decided to create alternative, more hopeful and supportive (in this case, more grateful) self-talk about the situation.

Here are some more examples of shifting one's negative self-talk toward gratitude (particularly about topics that are common as we age and about which it's easy to be negative):

Negative self-talk	Grateful alternative
"I have so much less energy than I did even 10 years ago."	"I'm grateful that I can still do yoga regularly and take long walks."
"It's depressing when friends my age die."	"I'm much more appreciative of the friends I still have."
"I miss having a respected job."	"I'm happy to have the time to pursue activities I love."
"I hate how society talks about old people."	"I'm glad the people I care about respect and love me—no matter how old I am!"

An important caveat: I'm not encouraging you to dismiss or ignore your negative feelings–all of the negative self-talk I noted above is perfectly legitimate; these aspects of getting old can be really difficult. It's healthy to feel your feelings, whatever they may be. And it's really healthy–and an important component of a great later life–to *also* be able to see the possibilities for gratitude, especially in difficult situations.

TRY IT

So now I encourage you to think of a couple of elements of your later life that bug you–things about which you regularly complain, either to yourself or to others. Below, write your self-talk about these things (as always, you can also do this activity at thenewoldbook.com).

Now, think about something for which you are (or can be) genuinely grateful in these same situations. Some aspects of each situation, difficult though it may be, that you find positive, or some positive thing that arises from the negative situation (like my interviewee who is losing his sight yet appreciates the opportunities that has created to deepen important relationships). Below, note the self-talk you'll use to acknowledge your gratitude:

My negative self-talk about current situations	Alternative grateful self-talk
1.	1.
2.	2.

3.	3.

If this approach appeals to you, keep playing with it. In a quiet moment, notice one thing you've been complaining about lately and recognize your negative self-talk about it (you can even write it down if you want). Do what you just did above: create a "grateful alternative"–something you can *also* say to yourself about the situation that seems true to you but is grateful vs. negative or "complainy."

Then, whenever that particular complaint comes up in your mind, you can give gratitude equal airtime in your self-talk. Notice how this makes you feel and if, over time, you're getting some of the "gratitude benefits" you hoped for.

Being Grateful About the Now

Another approach to developing a gratitude habit starts from the mindfulness we practiced in the previous chapter. As we discussed in that chapter, quite often, the things that worry us or make us mad, sad, anxious, or dissatisfied are things that haven't happened yet (and may not happen at all) or have already happened. In other words, they're not things that are happening at this moment. Even in a difficult, boring, or challenging situation, there are often interesting, fun, beautiful, or fascinating things occurring in the present moment–things for which we can be grateful.

Here's an example. Last year, my husband and I went through a very long, complicated and frustrating process of applying for a residency visa in Spain. We were on the final step–sitting in the office of immigration and naturalization waiting for our appointment to receive our "Tarjeta de Indentidad de Extranjero" (or TIE), the card that would make our residency in Spain legal–toward which we had been working for almost a year. I was nervous; anxious that something would go wrong or that my Spanish wouldn't be up to the challenge. I was going over and over everything we had already done and worrying about what we'd do if we ran into problems. I was not in the present moment, and I was not having a great experience.

I didn't like how I was feeling. Almost on a whim, I decided to be more present–and to be more grateful. I took a deep breath and refocused my attention in the moment. Then I looked at my dear husband and felt fortunate that we had both decided that this is what we wanted–it was so much easier and more fun to be on this adventure together. Then I noticed where I was: sitting in the middle of our new city of Oviedo–how grateful I felt that we had found such a lovely place to live that suited us so well. Then I noticed the people around us, speaking to each other in Spanish, and realized that I understood almost everything they were saying. I felt fortunate that my efforts to learn Spanish were working so well.

I had spent less than a minute refocusing my attention in the present moment and noticing some things for which I was genuinely grateful, but I immediately felt calmer, happier, more hopeful. We got called into the office a few minutes later, and everything turned out fine (I even got the lady behind the counter to crack a smile with my effusive thanks), and now we have our "TIEs." But for me, the best part of the experience was realizing the power of feeling grateful about the "now," even in an anxiety-inducing situation.

Now, I'm going to encourage you to do the same: to focus on some things for which you're grateful in this current moment. It could be something you see, hear, taste, smell, or feel. It could be a positive emotion you're having (yes, you can feel grateful to be happy, or curious, or energized).

As with the mindfulness exercises you did previously, make sure you'll be reasonably comfortable and undisturbed for the 5-10 minutes you'll be doing this exercise.

You'll simply be noting a few things for which you're genuinely grateful in the present moment.

You may discover a stream of "anti-grateful" thoughts in your head at the same time. For example, you might say to yourself, *I love that I get to hear the birdsong when I'm sitting here,* and your mind might also say to you, *That would be irritating if I heard it all the time,* or *I read somewhere there are fewer birds now because of climate change.*

Both those things may be true, but you can choose to put your focus back on feeling grateful at this particular moment. That's your goal in this "gratitude mindfulness" activity.

TRY IT

> Put this book aside and do the activity. Pick the book up again when you're done, in 5-10 minutes, and reflect on the following questions:
>
> - If you feel any differently than when you began the exercise, how would you describe the differences?
> - How easy or difficult was it to notice things in the moment for which to be grateful?
> - How could you make it easier for yourself to be grateful in the moment?

Then, after you've finished the activity, you can ramp up the benefits by noting your gratitude out loud. In her lovely book, *The Gratitude Diaries*, Janice Kaplan cites research showing that expressing your gratitude to others increases the benefits even more.[5] For example, if you noticed during this activity that you felt grateful about something that involves another person, tell them. It will make you feel even more grateful, and it will feel lovely to them as well.

Making Gratitude a Habit

So now you have some new tools for increasing your aspiration to be grateful, for managing your self-talk toward gratitude, and for being grateful in the moment. Let's use what you've already learned about making habits to use these tools consistently. As you may recall, in Chapter 7, I mentioned James Clear's *Atomic Habits*[6] and BJ Fogg's *Tiny Habits*[7]. Both authors recommend that you create new habits by focusing on small, easy changes that you can link to or build on pre-existing habits.

We've already got the small, easy change part right: shifting your self-talk toward gratitude and/or noticing elements of your current moment to be grateful for are both quick and easy. So, now, let's find a place to build gratitude into your existing habits.

Pick a habit you're already doing that gives you a bit of time to reflect–maybe when you're taking the dog for a walk or sitting with a cup of coffee after breakfast. Simply add in a few moments of acknowledging something for which you're grateful.

You might also leverage the power of committing to another person. Remember that people are much more likely to do things that they've told another person they're going to do. So, for instance, if you already have a regular time to get together with a friend or spouse–a morning walk or a review of the day while making dinner–agree that a bit of that time will also be spent sharing with each other things for which you're grateful.

My husband and I have made a habit like this: many evenings after dinner, we watch TV, but before we fire up the Google Play, we spend a couple of minutes sharing with each other what we've felt grateful for that day. It's a lovely, easy little habit, and it makes us both feel great (and loved, since one thing we often note feeling grateful for is each other).

TRY IT

Make a note to yourself, below or at thenewoldbook.com, what existing habit you'll link your new gratitude habit to:

> I'll take a few moments to feel grateful while I'm:

Remember, writing down a commitment also makes it more likely that you'll do it!

So, I hope these last three chapters have left you feeling both more able and more motivated to master your mindset, and that you're seeing what a valuable capability that is for someone who wants to create a great later life. It's especially important to remember that even as we age and may have less power in some ways—we may no longer have an influential job or the level of physical strength we once had—for most of us, our minds and hearts are as powerful, or more powerful, than ever. In the words of the American novelist Alice Walker: "The most common way people give up their power is by thinking they don't have any."

Now that you have the tools for building a hopeful, accurate, powerful frame of mind, let's talk about change.

> **THE BIG IDEA: Establishing a regular practice of being grateful feels wonderful and is an especially powerful tool for countering the challenges and difficulties of aging.**

[1] Allen, S. (2018). *Why is gratitude so hard for some people?* Greater Good Magazine. https://greatergood.berkeley.edu/article/item/why_is_gratitude_so_hard_for_so me_people

[2] Harvard Health Publishing. (2021). *Giving thanks can make you happier.* Harvard Medical School. https://www.health.harvard.edu/healthbeat/giving-thanks-can-make-you-happier#:~:text=In%20positive%20psychology%20research%2C%20gratitude,expr ess%20gratitude%20in%20multiple%20ways

[3] Ethos. (2021). The importance of gratitude for senior health. https://www.ethoscare.org/news/the-benefits-of-gratitude-in-older-adults

[4] Morin, A. (2015). *7 Scientifically proven benefits of gratitude.* Psychology Today. https://www.psychologytoday.com/us/blog/what-mentally-strong-people-dont-do/201504/7-scientifically-proven-benefits-of-gratitude

[5] Kaplan, J. (2016). *The gratitude diaries.* Dutton

[6] Clear, J. (2018). Atomic habits: An easy and proven way to build good habits and break bad ones. First Edition. Avery

[7] Fogg, BJ. (2019). Tiny habits: The tiny changes that change everything. Harvest

Principle III:
Get Good at Change

10. How We Go Through Change

"It's not about standing still and becoming safe. If anybody wants to keep creating, they have to be about change." —Miles Davis

There seems to be a widespread belief that older people's lives are more or less unchanging–even stagnant. After all, we're generally not juggling jobs and kids and aging parents, and we may be more comfortable financially, and so not having to put so much energy into worrying about that.

You see this belief reflected in online quizzes and polls that ask about your age. They go by decade until the final category of "60+" or "over 65"–implying that everyone over 60 or 65 is pretty much the same, whether they're 68 or 98.

My experience, though, and that of most people I interviewed for this book, is exactly the opposite. We're finding that later life is chock full of change, and that it's often of the most challenging kind: change that's imposed upon us rather than chosen by us. And then, of course, there's the biggest and most daunting change we face in later life: we are all going to die. And it's going to be in 20 or 30 years, rather than 60 or 70. Every single person I know who's in the last third of their life has experienced the deaths of close friends and family members: parents, siblings, colleagues, school friends. We talked about this earlier, in the "terrifying" chapter, but it deserves to be mentioned again here; it's the ultimate change, and one over which, in the end, we have zero control.

We're also dealing with a variety of lesser changes. There are the shifts in our physical capabilities and our health conditions, even if we're fortunate enough to be basically healthy. Then, there's the ripple effect

143

of all the accommodations and alterations in habit and approach that result from these changes in our health. Things we used to find easy and did without even thinking can become challenging or impossible. My husband, an amazing handyman, no longer feels safe balancing at the top of a ladder. Should he brave it anyway? Look for a different, more stable kind of ladder? Hire somebody to do ladder-top tasks? Decide they don't really need to be done? In other words, each change creates its own cascade of decision and action, and most of us are dealing with multiple changes of this kind.

Then, too, we're dealing with changes in our identity. For many of us, our work life has been a big part of that identity, and retirement (or even semi-retirement) changes how others see us and how we see ourselves. I spent 35 years introducing myself as the founding partner and CEO of my company, Proteus International. I'm no longer the CEO, and though I'm still the founder, that becomes a different role now that I'm no longer actively managing the company. Proteus will always be a part of who I am—but my relationship with it has changed and will continue to change, in ways that affect how I see myself, how I live my life, how I interact with others, and how they view and interact with me.

There are changes in our non-work identities, as well. For example, who you are as a parent of teenagers or even young adults is very different from who you are as a parent of middle-aged people with mortgages and teenagers of their own. Many older people are also getting divorced these days, and it can be a profound alteration in your sense of self when you're no longer married to the same person after 20, 30, or 40 years. And for many of us, what we do with our leisure time may also change as we get older (pickleball instead of tennis, long nature walks instead of rock climbing), and that may affect not only how we spend our time but how we see ourselves.

And finally, there are the changes in how society sees and relates to you as an old person. I talked about this quite a bit in the first couple of chapters: it's a big change for a lot of us to recognize that many of the people we deal with on a daily basis, both personally and professionally, assume different and often less positive things about us because we're older–about our capabilities, our intelligence, our interests and even our usefulness (or the lack thereof).

Many seniors try to fight back against these changes by striving to keep the circumstances of their lives artificially the same.[1] I can't tell you how many stories I've heard of parents or grandparents who want to stay in the same house (even though it's too big, expensive and hard to take care of); vacation in the same place and with the same people; eat the same food at the same time in the same place; watch the same TV shows; wear the same clothes; have the same conversations. And, more troubling, I've been told about older people who refuse to address medical issues because they don't want to acknowledge that their physical condition may be changing, or those who avoid using new, helpful technology because it's "not what they're used to."

To top it all off, change in general, for everyone, is speeding up and getting more disruptive. I previously mentioned my last book, *Change from the Inside Out*, where I make this case in-depth: that our world is changing ever more quickly and that most human beings find change difficult–especially when it's not their idea.

So Here We Are

We live in a world that is changing every day, and our lives as older people–contrary to popular belief–are also changing in profound and often difficult ways. To craft a great later life for ourselves, we have to get good at change...perhaps even better at it than younger people. And thus, the third principle of the book.

Over the next three chapters, I'm going to offer you lots of insights and tools that will support you to keep changing and growing as you age so that you can continue to craft the later life that will most satisfy you. First, though, I want to give you a grounding in how human beings go through change.

Discovering how the process of going through change happens was the big ah-ha for me at the core of *Change from the Inside Out*, and if you want a more in-depth discussion–and one focused more on organizations–you're welcome to check it out.[2] For our purposes here, I'm going to focus on the elements that are universally applicable, and especially those that relate to us as older adults.

Why Is Change So Hard?

I've noted above many ways we, as older people, try to resist change, but it's not just us–externally imposed change is difficult for most people. In writing *Change from the Inside Out*, this was the main code I wanted to crack. I figured if I could understand why change is so hard for most people, I'd be better able to help people overcome that difficulty.

As I researched and talked to people about change and how they felt about it, I understood something very important about why change–especially externally-imposed change–is so hard for us. I realized that until the past few hundred years, most people's lives were hugely more predictable and stable than our lives are today. People generally were born, grew up, and died in one place, and it was usually where their parents and grandparents had been born, grown up, and died. People most often did the same work their parents and grandparents had done: they were farmers or builders, soldiers or brewers, and they knew what was expected of them in that work because they grew up watching and learning from those previous generations. No big surprises or changes there, generally speaking. People also belonged to the same church as their parents and grandparents, ate the same food, went to the same market, had the same neighbors, wore the same kind of clothing, and had the same relationships with the local government or ruler. Very little changed, day to day.

Major, unexpected change was unusual, and–this is important to note–that kind of change was generally a very bad thing: a war, a plague, a flood, a famine. And when one of these dreadful, disruptive, deadly changes arrived, the main thing everyone wanted to do was to get back to the status quo–where there wasn't a war, flood, famine, or plague–as soon as they could.

So, looking at our history as humans, you can see that over many thousands of years, we learned to see externally-imposed change as bad and scary, and to do everything in our power, when confronted with those terrifying changes, to get back to the "safe" pre-change state as quickly as possible. In fact, this became a survival mechanism: those people who were best at figuring out how to return to a non-flood, famine, war, or plague situation as quickly as possible were those who tended to live and reproduce.

Given all this, it's no wonder that when something important looks like it's going to change in ways that we haven't instigated (our health, where we live, what we do day-to-day), we don't like it. We want things to stay the same.

So, How Do We Get Better at Changing?

I suspect you won't be surprised to know that I'm about to offer you some help with this problem. As I noted, when I was starting to write my previous book about change, I figured that if I could get clear about what happens within an individual, emotionally and psychologically, when that person *successfully* goes through a change, my colleagues and

I would be better able to support people (ourselves included) to go through change more easily.

And the result of all that thinking and research was (voilà) that we came to understand the process we now call The Change Arc. It describes how humans go through change:

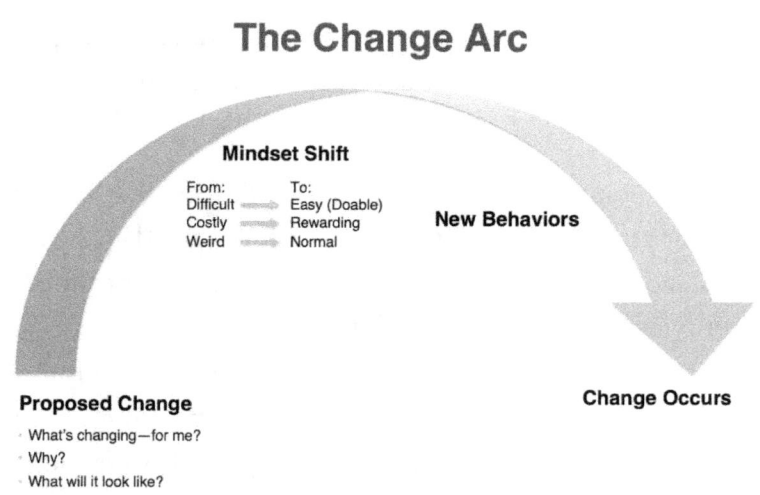

The Change Arc

Mindset Shift

From: To:
Difficult ➝ Easy (Doable)
Costly ➝ Rewarding
Weird ➝ Normal

New Behaviors

Proposed Change
· What's changing—for me?
· Why?
· What will it look like?

Change Occurs

Here's how this works. When any kind of a change is first proposed (or imposed), we almost always have three questions about the change. These questions are remarkably predictable: we tend to have them no matter how big or small the change, and no matter whether the change might seem at first glance to be largely positive or largely negative.

We want to know, first of all, how the change will affect us personally; in other words, *what will be changing for us*. In doing this research, we came to see this question as being a part of that ancient wiring I talked about earlier. In posing this question, we're trying to figure out how dangerous and disruptive this change will be for us individually so that we're prepared to respond (usually by going back to the pre-change state).

Then, we want some reasons: *Why is the change happening?* Since we generally prefer the status quo (unless the change was our idea), with this question we're kind of saying, "OK, if you expect me to accept this change, there better be a damn good reason for it."

Finally, we want to know *what our world will look like once the change has been made.* Interestingly, one of the things I discovered in researching the *Change* book was that a lot of psychologists and psychiatrists believe that our deepest fear is fear of the unknown.[3] So one of the scariest things about an externally imposed change is that it's a walk into the unknown...and we're not OK with that. We really want to know what we're getting ourselves into if we accept this change.

Plus, we already think it's going to be bad...

Now, as we're asking these questions, it turns out that our experience is further complicated by the fact that we're quite often filtering the responses we get through our negative beliefs and expectations about change. In fact, we found in our research that the most common beliefs people have about change–any change–are that it will be *difficult, costly* and *weird.*

Difficult means "I don't know how to do this, and/or other people are going to make it hard for me." *Costly* means "it's going to take from me things I value." (This can be things like time or money–but it's even more likely that we think the change is going to take away more essential, intrinsically valuable things like identity, relationships, respect, freedom, dignity.) *Weird* means unnatural, as in "This is not how I see myself," or "This is not how I like things to be."

And all this comes from our historically negative wiring about change: remember, in ages past, most unexpected change *was* difficult, costly (often costing our lives!), and weird. And here in the twenty-first century, we still tend to expect that any newly-arisen change will be difficult, costly, and weird. So, you can imagine that even if we're getting pretty good answers to our initial three questions (about what the change means for us, why it's happening, and what it will look like when it's done), we're still not going to be very open to or happy about the change. We are, in fact, likely to feel angry, sad, overwhelmed, demoralized, or resentful. Those negative feelings and expectations can make the change much more painful and difficult to navigate.

But Here's the Good News...

As we clarified this challenging truth about most people's approach to change, though, we also stumbled upon the solution. We saw that when someone *was* able to make a change, it was rarely because something external shifted; it was almost always because that person's mindset changed, and it changed in a predictable and specific way.

You'll notice that the middle part of the Change Arc, above, is labelled "Mindshift Shift"–and that, dear reader, is the heart of the process. We learned that when someone's mindset shifts from thinking that a change is going to be difficult, costly and weird, to thinking that it *could be* easy (or at least doable), rewarding and normal–then that person will be able and willing to make the change, and the change can happen as easily and (relatively) painlessly as possible. That's the shift shown on the Change Arc above. And one important aspect of what we discovered is that the critical mindset shift is what I just noted: when a person goes from believing that the change will be bad (difficult, costly and weird) to thinking that *it could be* OK (easy/doable, rewarding, normal), they are generally able to make the change. In other words, to get the benefits of this mindset shift, you don't even have to be convinced that the change will be a positive thing–just open to the possibility.

What does this "easy, rewarding and normal" frame look like in terms of a change? *Easy*–or if not easy, at least *doable*–means thinking that you could be capable of learning or doing what's needed to deal with or accept this change. It means believing you could be able to handle it: that it won't be too much for you.

Rewarding simply means that you think it could give you some valuable things or have some positive outcomes: that it won't only take things away from you.

And *normal* means it could come to seem regular and even natural–not strange and uncomfortable.

I can't overstate how fundamental this discovery was. When I understood this truth, I felt like Archimedes in the bathtub; I almost yelled, "Eureka!" Let me explain my excitement: This means that getting good at change is almost entirely within our control, because the main skill required is learning how to shift our mindset about change. And we all have control–or can learn to have control–over our own thoughts.

And, as I'm pleased to remind you, controlling your thoughts–your self-talk–is something we've been focusing on together for the past three chapters. So, break out the champagne: This is simply a different application of the skill of managing your self-talk.

Managing Your Self-Talk About Change

Our belief that an imposed-on-us change is going to be difficult, costly and weird is reflected in how we talk to ourselves about it. So, let's apply the approach you've learned for shifting your self-talk to this situation: changing how you talk to yourself about change. The four steps are exactly the same:

- *recognize* your unhelpful self-talk about the change (that proposes it's going to be difficult, costly and weird),
- *record* it to separate yourself from it a bit,

- *revise* it to acknowledge the possibility of the change being easy/doable, rewarding and normal, in a way that's believable by you, and then,
- *repeat* your more change-supportive self-talk as needed.

An example. Let's say that you've just discovered that an unwelcome change has intruded itself into your life: you've developed a mild case of something called Essential Tremor Disorder, a very common condition in older people, where different parts of your body (most often hands or feet, but often the neck or head) develop a fine tremor. It's more common the older you get; it's estimated that almost 1 in 10 people over 80 may have it.[4]

I've been dealing with this myself over the past year (it started first in my neck), so this is a true-life example. I noticed that my initial self-talk about it was definitely of the difficult, costly and weird variety, e.g.: *Oh, I hate this, it feels so strange (*weird*). I won't be able to deal with it (*difficult*), and it's going to make me seem like an old lady (*costly*)!*

I wrote out the preceding self-talk, which had the usual effect I experience when writing down my negative self-talk: it made me think, *Wow, that sucks. I don't want to think like that. I don't even really believe it.*

So, then I revised my self-talk toward the possibility that this change *could be* doable, bring some reward, and be somewhat normal:

Difficult: *I won't be able to deal with this*

to

Doable: *I don't know how to deal with it yet, so let me do some research. I'm sure there are simple ways to manage it.*

Costly: *It's going to make me seem like an old lady*

to

Rewarding: *I wonder if it could make me more conscious of when I'm stressed and of how I'm holding my body?*

Weird: *This is so strange*

to

Normal: *I need to find out how other people deal with this and how common it is.*

What happened when I shifted my self-talk in this way? I started to do the things my self-talk encouraged me to do (did some research, talked to some other people, got more aware of what was happening in my body), and as a result, I was able to accept and accommodate the change. I've incorporated the fact of this slight neurological disorder into my yoga practice (it turns out yoga is a very good thing for ET) and into how I manage my stress. Interestingly, it turns out that ET is a good early warning system for stress–my neck tremor gets much worse when I'm experiencing psychological stress, so if my neck is trembling, it's a good signal for me to note what's stressing me out and deal with it. I'm thinking of that as a slight reward.

In other words, shifting my mindset allowed me to continue moving along the Change Arc: I started doing the new behaviors the change required, and the change–my acceptance of and accommodation to the condition–occurred.

More importantly, the change occurred without me kicking and screaming (mentally) about it. It has been fairly simple and non-disruptive, given my new knowledge and the steps I was able to take to address it. Ironically, what I now know about ET and stress leads me to believe that my condition probably would have become much worse if I had stayed negative and unhappy about it...the kind of vicious cycle that often happens when we resist a change.

TRY IT

I encourage you to test this out with some change that you're dealing with at the moment. It could be anything, but it will be most useful to pick a change with which you're having a hard time:

My self-talk proposing that this change is/will be difficult, costly, and weird:	Easy/doable, rewarding, normal alternative self-talk:
1.	1.
2.	2.
3.	3.

If that was easy for you, congratulations! Now comes the "repeat" part of the skill of managing your self-talk: when your mind offers (again) your original, anti-change self-talk, just substitute your revised, more change-capable self-talk, and note what happens. I suspect it will trend you in the direction of doing the behaviors required by the change, that is, of moving you along the Change Arc.

What If It Didn't Work?

If, on the other hand, you found that activity difficult or even impossible—that you simply couldn't imagine saying to yourself that the change you're dealing with could be doable (let alone easy), or rewarding, or normal, I have something else for you to try.

We may need to address your change resistance on the level of belief rather than just on the level of self-talk. That's necessary if your self-talk represents a truly negative anti-change belief.

Here's what I mean by that. As I've already noted, often our self-talk doesn't reflect our true beliefs; it's just habitual. For example, I've mentioned that when I write down my negative self-talk, my immediate response is often some version of, "Wow, I don't even really believe that." In cases like that, when you change your self-talk, you're simply better aligning your mental monologue with your actual beliefs about the situation, and that change in your self-talk is likely to work very well.

But what if your negative self-talk *is* reflecting your current beliefs? What if you actually believe your negative self-talk about a change you're facing? In other words, what do you do in a change situation if you truly think that this change *will* be difficult, costly and weird?

Then you need to work first on changing your beliefs.

Getting Curious About A Change

Let me start by reminding you that it's not surprising if you have strong negative beliefs about a change. Remember all our historical programming that tells us change is scary, bad and disruptive? Add to that any personal negative experiences you've had with change (that only serve to reinforce that historical wiring). And on top of that, there's the fact that a lot of the changes we have to deal with as older people aren't fun, positive (getting your hip replaced is no one's idea of a good time), or optional. So firmly believing that a particular unavoidable change is going to suck–is going to be difficult, costly and weird–is understandable.

And if you can learn to change even those firmly held, seemingly reasonable negative beliefs about particular changes, it will make your life a lot more pleasant and less stressful.

We'll use the power of curiosity to question your current beliefs about the change you're dealing with. I've talked and written a lot about curiosity as a skill. Curiosity is jet fuel for learning[5]–and we'll talk about it a lot more in the coming chapters about modifying gracefully and acquiring new skills and knowledge. For now, though, we'll take advantage of one of the wonderful things about curiosity: it's a marvelous tool for questioning the status quo.

If you think about it, being curious is a state of questioning. When we're curious, we want to know, or learn, or find out more–we're not simply accepting our current understanding. So, then, how about if you questioned your beliefs about this change being difficult, costly and weird; questioned them with genuine curiosity about the possibility of an alternative set of beliefs?

A great curiosity-based question often starts with "How can/could...?" We already talked about using "How can I" questions in chapter 4 when we were envisioning our best later life. (You might remember that I asked myself the question, "How can I become what comes after the butterfly?") We've seen over and over that "How can/could...?" questions encourage people to challenge their assumptions and to think more reflectively about possibilities rather than simply concluding what they already believe.

Let's use a very common example to show how using "How can/could...?" questions can help you shift your beliefs about a change you're facing. Imagine you have to get a hip replacement, and you truly believe that it's going to be extremely difficult, costly, and weird. In this situation, you could try asking yourself:

How could this situation be easier to handle? How could I make it more doable?

How could getting my hip replaced be rewarding? What positive outcomes might there be?

How can I make this whole process more normal and less weird?

Here's how it might look to ask and answer those questions about a hip replacement:

How could this situation be easier to handle? How could I make it more doable?

I'll do some research so I know what to expect and ensure I'm mentally and physically set up to support the best and fastest possible recovery.

How could getting my hip replaced be rewarding? What positive outcomes might there be?

I've heard that the kind of pain I've been experiencing goes away almost immediately. And the doctor says I should be able to get back out on the nature trails within a few months–which I haven't been able to do for the past year or two.

How can I make this whole process more normal and less weird?

I think talking to people I like and respect who have had this procedure–either in-person or online–will help me see this as something common that millions of people go through. And being able to walk without pain will definitely be more normal!

Asking "How can/could...?" questions is a kind of nicely sneaky way to get past your firm anti-change beliefs. Asking these questions engages your brain gently in imagining a possible alternative, and often, before you know it, you've come up with some answers that show you your beliefs aren't entirely accurate. When I've used this approach with people in the past, they often say things like, "Well, I guess if I did X, it might make this a lot easier," or "It's possible that this could have Y positive outcome." It's almost like we're reluctant to acknowledge that a tough change could be OK–but in looking for the answers to "How can/could...?" questions, you just can't help doing it.

TRY IT

So, if you're finding that your anti-change beliefs are strong in this instance, here's your chance to try questioning them:

Look back at the difficult/costly/weird self-talk you noted above about this change in your life and ask:

- How could I make this change easier or more doable for myself?

- How could this change have some positive outcomes?

- How could I make this change more normal and less weird?

If your anti-change beliefs in this instance are particularly strong or stuck, you may need to be patient with yourself and be willing to ask yourself these questions a couple of times. That is, the first answer you get from yourself might be along the lines of, "I can't! There's nothing I can do to make this easier."

In that case, I encourage you to take a deep breath and talk back to yourself. You could say something like, "OK. But if there was some way I *could* make it easier, what might that be?"

Remember, it's in your best interests to become more fluent with and less upset by change–especially necessary and unavoidable change. I assure you that nothing bad will happen if you soften your negative beliefs about change. A few years ago, I did this exercise with one of the executives I was coaching. He noted, "You know, I thought I was protecting myself by believing that change was always hard–almost like it couldn't blindside me if I expected it to be terrible. But I'm seeing now that I've just been making everything a lot more difficult for myself, assuming the worst. This allows me to apply my problem-solving skills to make change as smooth and relatively painless as possible."

Exactly.

Making Change-Capability a Habit

We've worked a lot over the past few chapters on making habits of the skills and tools we've been discussing. So, I'll just remind you of these key habit-building approaches:

- **Find the personal benefits**
- **Envision a future where you're reaping those benefits**
- **Connect your new habit to an existing habit**

And if you want to remind yourself of how these approaches work, I invite you to go back to Chapter 7, where we first started talking about how to make managing our self-talk a habit.

And One Last Thing...

I was talking about this chapter to a friend recently, and he said, "This is all well and good–but what about those changes that really *are* horrible? The death of a spouse or sibling, a terminal illness, the loss of your sight or hearing? You can't just magically think that stuff is going to be easy, rewarding and normal."

I agree a thousand percent. Some things–and they can happen at any point in our lives but seem to come with greater frequency when we're older–are simply dreadful, and there's no way around it. When a horrible change happens, it's normal and healthy to rage and grieve. Pretending everything is OK right away is just another form of avoiding change.

And I submit to you that what I'm saying still applies. When you're ready to move on and figure out how to live your life as well as possible given a negative change, this mindset shift approach can be very helpful. I would remind you, as a great, real-life example, of my interviewee who is losing his sight. He has figured out how to make it doable, with a combination of assistive technology and help from his wife and others; he's noted the reward of deeper relationships and conversations with those he cares about; and he talked to me about how it's become his new normal–not what he would have preferred, but what he has now accepted as his reality.

Permanently rejecting, resisting and raging against an unavoidable change benefits no one, least of all you. Consistently working to shift your mindset about change toward acceptance and solution-orientation is the best way to continue to craft your best later life, through whatever may come.

Now, let's talk about what comes next. Once you've shifted your mindset, how do you shift your behavior and habits? We call it "modifying gracefully"....

THE BIG IDEA: Getting good at change is a key skill for anyone these days–but is especially important to thrive through the changes that come with age. AND it's learnable.

---

[1] National Research Council (US) Committee on Aging Frontiers in Social Psychology, Personality, and Adult Developmental Psychology. (2006). Motivation and behavioral change. In *When I'm 64. Carstensen, L. L., Hartel, C. R. (Eds.)*. Washington (DC): National Academies Press (US). https://www.ncbi.nlm.nih.gov/books/NBK83771/

[2] Andersen, E. (2021). Change from the inside out: Making you, your team and your organization change-capable. Berrett-Koehler Publishers

[3] Carleton, R. N. (2016). Fear of the unknown: One fear to rule them all? *Journal of anxiety disorders*, *41*, 5-21. https://www.sciencedirect.com/science/article/pii/S0887618516300469#.

[4] Song, P., Zhang, Y., Zha, M., Yang, Q., Ye, X., Yi, Q., & Rudan, I. (2021). The global prevalence of essential tremor, with emphasis on age and sex: a meta-analysis. *Journal of global health*, *11*, 04028. https://www.ncbi.nlm.nih.gov/pmc/articles/PMC8035980/

[5] Andersen, E. (2016). Be bad first: Get good at things fast to stay ready for the future. Routledge

11. Modify Gracefully

"Aging gracefully means being flexible, being open, allowing change, enjoying change and loving yourself." —Wendy Whelan

Once, about 20 years ago, I was in Macy's in Manhattan, looking through the handbags on a sale table. A hand entered my field of vision, a very old hand, judging by the liver spots, wrinkles, and nearly transparent skin showing blue veins beneath. She pointed to a purse I was looking at and said (in her very old person's slightly tremulous voice). "That one's nice, isn't it?" I turned to respond and almost jumped in shock when I saw the rest of her.

Despite the evidence of her voice and hands, she was doing her best to pretend she was 25. Thinning hair dyed dark brown and fluffed over her skull; lots of dramatic eye make-up and red lipstick; a mini-skirt and tight, brightly colored sweater; very high heels. Her choice, of course, and if that's how she felt best, more power to her. But to me, it was a perfect example of not modifying gracefully, and I vowed at that moment that when I got old, I wouldn't try to hold on to my youth in that way.

So now I am old, and I'm on a daily quest to figure out how to modify gracefully. Graceful is defined as "characterized by elegance or beauty of form, manner, movement or speech." So, modifying gracefully as you age means figuring out how to change as necessary in an elegant, beautiful way that feels comfortable and relatively easy to you, not stiff, unyielding, or difficult. At the same time, we don't need to limit ourselves unnecessarily just because we're aging: we can modify well and appropriately, and in a way that works best for us–that, to me, is another aspect of grace.

Change Is Hard...Yet Again

I've just spent a whole chapter telling you how hard it is for us to change, especially when the change isn't our idea. So, it shouldn't be much of a surprise to find out that making necessary behavioral changes as older people can be really challenging. When we're faced with the need not only to change our mindset about a needed change but then actually to do something differently, it can be hard on lots of levels. In a recent report outlined in The Gerontologist[1], based on behavior change workshops done with older adults, scientists found that the obstacles to doing things differently for old people can include both external environmental factors–physical, social, health care or financial–and internal behavioral factors, like beliefs, knowledge, habits, constraints, goals and desires, self-efficacy and even brain chemistry. Yikes.

And hidden in that pile of obstacles, buried somewhere between "social environment," "beliefs," and "habits," is what I've seen as the key obstacle: loss of identity. This lives in the "costly" bucket of how we think about change: we're concerned that making changes to our lives is going to cost us our preferred identity, both with ourselves and with others.

A friend of mine in Spain told me about her mom, who is in her late 80s. She was very active until about 18 months ago, when she fell and broke her hip. (Falling is the leading cause of injury in adults 65 and older[2].) Fortunately, her hip healed without complication, but even when she was able, she refused to leave her apartment because she still needed to use a walker, and she didn't want "her friends to see her as some crippled old person." As a result, she is quickly losing conditioning and becoming depressed; her family and her doctor are concerned about her long-term prognosis. Her refusal to accept the new behaviors required by this change, a change that is, from her point of view, costing her identity as an active and vital person, may ultimately cost her life.

You Have Tools!

Fortunately, all the tools we've discussed throughout our time together will be valuable in learning to make the modifications that aging will require of you. To recap:

- *Envisioning the future* you want to create for yourself will help you stay focused on what's most important to you, even as your circumstances require modification,
- Knowing how to *make it happen* will support you in figuring out the necessary accommodations and building your aspiration to do so,
- Building and *leading your* supportive *crew* can help to minimize external obstacles to changing,
- *Managing your self-talk* is key to creating an internal environment that supports modifying gracefully,
- Staying *mindful* and *grateful* will allow you to focus on joy, beauty and what's working in your life, even as you need to change,
- Perhaps most importantly, understanding *how we go through change* gives you a simple, powerful frame for deciding how best to modify when needed.

Making It Less Difficult, Costly and Weird...

Let's start there, continuing the approach we experimented with in the last chapter, applying "How can/could...?" questions. Now, we'll use them to decide how to modify some part of your life to make it easier, more rewarding, and normal.

I'd like to use as an example a very personal part of our lives: our sexuality as older adults. I'm choosing this because it's an area where modification is almost inevitable (75-year-old sex is very different, for most people, from 35-year-old sex). The sexual ageism that exists in most cultures around the world makes modifying this part of our lives even more challenging. A recent article on this topic noted that "today's society is still significantly permeated by an 'ageing-phobic' vision that unfairly tends to depict and lump all people aged 65 or older into a group of old, frail, undesirable, and asexual beings, separate from the rest of society."[3] When society at large and even we ourselves think that we aren't sexual beings as older people[4], it creates additional mental, emotional and even physiological obstacles to making necessary changes in this part of our lives.

I want to share the positive experience of one of my interviewees and her husband, just to show you how graceful modification is possible even in a realm like sexuality that's fraught with obstacles. This couple had always had a really satisfying, fun and intimate sex life until their early 70s, when the husband began to experience severe erectile dysfunction. He had used Cialis for some years, and it had worked well, but over time, it stopped working, and he wasn't able to get an erection. He tried Viagra and even an injectable drug, but nothing worked. His libido was still high, and he could have orgasms; he just wasn't able to get an erection.

For many months after this, the couple's sexual relationship consisted of lots of cuddling and kissing, mutual masturbation, fellatio and cunnilingus–but they missed having intercourse.

Because they have very good communication and were willing and able to talk about the situation, they found themselves asking a key question: *"How can we find a satisfying alternative to 'regular' sexual intercourse?"* In other words, they started looking for a way to make it more easy, rewarding, and normal to have sex without an erect penis.

The husband hit on the idea of using a strap-on dildo; the wife was more than willing to try it. After a period of trial and error (it turned out there are lots of options available on the market), they settled on a model that felt comfortable to both of them and was easy for the husband to incorporate into their sex play. She told me that they now find it fun and sexually satisfying–and confided that they're proud of how they figured out how to shift their approach in a way that worked. "We're also, honestly, stoked that we're still so focused on having a great sex life in our 70s–and for the rest of our lives," she added, grinning. "It's kind of a private 'screw you' to anybody who thinks old people aren't sexual."

You can tell by what she shared with me that they've addressed a change that really was *difficult* (something they loved became impossible to do), *costly* (it was taking away something they enjoyed and identified with), and *weird* (it felt unnatural not to be able to have intercourse). They modified gracefully to make the situation more *easy* (this is a comfortable and simple alternative for both of them), *rewarding* (this is fun and sexually satisfying–and supports their identity as sexual beings), and *normal* (this way of having intercourse has become their new "regular"). Success.

Another example...

Let's look at making another modification toward easy, rewarding and normal using "How can/could...?" questions. We'll focus on the situation my friend's mom is in, where she needs to use a walker to get around (at least for the time being) after her hip fracture. What would happen if, instead of rejecting the change, she asked the three "How can/could...?" questions to figure out how best to modify:

- *How can I make this change easier or more doable for myself?*
- *How could this change have some positive outcomes?*
- *How can I make this change more normal and less weird?*

Here are some possible answers:

How can I make this change easier or doable for myself? I could start by having my daughter drive me in her car to take walks in places where I don't know anybody, so I won't feel embarrassed. Also, I could find out from the doctor how I can get strong enough not to use the walker–a cane would seem better.

How could this change have some positive outcome? My grandkids have offered to go on walks with me, and I don't see them as much as I'd like; this could be a way to spend time together. Also, my friend Carmen is in a wheelchair now, and we could bond over this–complaining is bonding!

How can I make this change more normal and less weird? If I accept that this is what's happening right now, I'll get used to it. And I guess if it doesn't seem weird to me, it probably won't seem weird to other people.

You'll notice that using this approach doesn't require you to be super-positive or cheerleader-ish–just to be open to the possibility that needed modification *could* be easy, rewarding and normal.

Knowing When You Need to Modify

Before we practice this (you knew I would make you practice, right?), let's talk about another important element that leads to not modifying when necessary: a lack of accurate self-awareness. In the early 2000s, my mom was becoming a pretty dangerous driver; her reflexes were slowing way down, and she would get confused and anxious in fast-moving traffic situations. None of us knew how to talk to her about it because she insisted that she was just fine and, in fact, "a much better driver than most of those idiots out there." She only acknowledged the situation had changed when my older sister told her she didn't feel safe having Mom drive her kids–Mom's grandkids. It was a very hard conversation for my sister to have, but it was necessary.

My mom was carrying an outdated version of herself as a driver. That's what I mean by a lack of accurate self-awareness. We often fail to modify as we age because we don't see ourselves as we are, but as we used to be, or as we want to be.

How Can You See Yourself Clearly?

This lack of accurate self-awareness isn't just a later-life problem. Most human beings have big blind spots about themselves–and we tend, unfortunately, to see ourselves least clearly in the areas that are most important to us.

I've mentioned one of my previous books, *Be Bad First*, which focuses on how to learn new things easily and well. And it turns out that a key mental skill for being a great learner is *neutral self-awareness*. It's very hard to learn anything unless you can be accurate about where you're starting from. For example, we all know people who think they're great at something and aren't–and those people tend to be very resistant to hearing about how they might improve in that area because they think they're already stellar.

If you think about it, figuring out how to modify gracefully is just a different kind of learning challenge: you need to learn how to do something in a new way that works in your current circumstances (like my interviewees and their sexuality). Therefore, you need to be clear about where you're starting from.

The key to neutral, accurate self-awareness is being able to be a *fair witness* about yourself. You may remember that I introduced this concept of being a fair witness in Chapter 4, when we discussed being accurate regarding your current state as a preparation for creating your later life vision.

Because fair witnessing means being as objective and accurate as possible, working on becoming a Fair Witness of yourself is the best way I know to increase your level of neutral self-awareness, and thereby expand your ability to learn new things well and quickly.

Here's the problem with this: as I noted earlier, the more important something is to you, and therefore the more emotionally attached you are to it, the more difficult it is to be fully objective about it. That means it can be challenging to 'fair witness' your changing circumstances and capabilities as you age, as well as your feelings about them. I'm sure you've noticed, for example, how much easier it is to see someone else's problems clearly and to give them good advice than it is to see your own problems and the best solutions to them.

Remember that older lady I mentioned at the beginning of the chapter? Now, it's possible that she was 100% self-aware and was making her stylistic choices with full consciousness–but I doubt it. It was more likely that she simply wasn't being a fair witness about herself and that it was important to her to continue to see herself as a young woman. That's called emotional attachment.

Fortunately, this rather demanding and often uncomfortable task of becoming your own fair witness requires a skill you already know: it's all about revising your self-talk in a specific way. Here's how it works:

Becoming your own fair witness:

- **Select an area of your life where you suspect you may need to change**
- **Recognize/record your self-talk about your own circumstances and capabilities in this area.**
- **Then ask yourself, "Is my self-talk accurate?"**
- **Where you're unsure, ask, "What facts do I have about myself in this area?"**
- **Revise your self-talk to be more accurate based on your answers.**

Let's imagine, for instance, that you've been an avid tennis player for many years, and you've noticed lately that it seems harder on your body than it used to be. You tune in to your self-talk about it and realize that you're telling yourself *I'm fine, I just need to power through. I don't want to be a wimp just because I'm getting old.*

So you ask yourself, "Is my self-talk accurate?"

If you let yourself be honest, your reflection on the accuracy of your self-talk will likely be something like: "I'm not sure 'powering through' is the smartest response. And is thinking about a less demanding alternative 'being a wimp'? I'm not sure that's true."

Since you believe your self-talk probably isn't accurate, but you're not sure, you can look for more facts. This might mean talking to your doctor or physical therapist about whether tennis is still a healthy activity for you and doing some research about similar but less demanding sports (pickleball, ping pong, or padel, for instance).

After talking to your service providers and doing your research, you might decide to revise your self-talk to something like: *I want to support and take great care of my body as it is now while still having fun and getting good exercise.*

And that's a perfect starting point for modifying gracefully.

Where and How Will You Modify?

Now, let's put this all together. I encourage you to pick an area of your life that you think you might need to modify. (This activity will be even more impactful if you're brave enough to pick an area where you suspect you've been actively resisting modification–perhaps where others have been telling you it's time to contemplate a change and where you've been defending your refusal to change.)

First, we'll focus on helping you become more of a fair witness of yourself in this area.

TRY IT

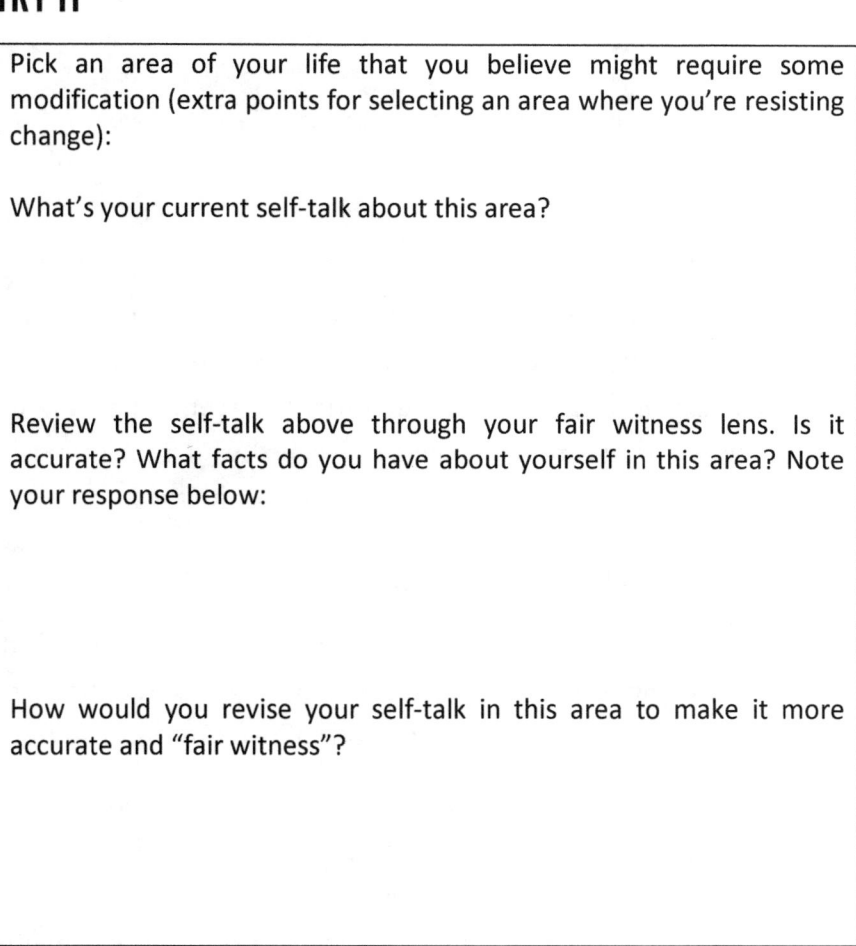

Pick an area of your life that you believe might require some modification (extra points for selecting an area where you're resisting change):

What's your current self-talk about this area?

Review the self-talk above through your fair witness lens. Is it accurate? What facts do you have about yourself in this area? Note your response below:

How would you revise your self-talk in this area to make it more accurate and "fair witness"?

Now that you've increased your self-awareness in this area and made it more neutral and accurate, you can figure out how to modify in a way that works for you by asking the three "How can/could...?" questions:

Reflecting on this area of your life, ask:

- How can I make this change easier or more doable for myself?

- How could this change have some positive outcomes?

- How can I make this change more normal and less weird?

The good news is that when you modify in this way, by starting on the level of your self-talk and revising it to be more accurate, it's more likely that you'll carry through with the modifications you come up with. And as you now know, when your beliefs are aligned with your proposed actions, you're much more likely to carry through with them.

And if this doesn't work right away...

As always with these activities, the proof is in the pudding. If you find, over the next few weeks, that you're *not* making the modifications you've proposed above, it's probably for one of two reasons.

It may be that you're still holding on to your previous "I'm good the way I am" self-talk–and therefore not believing that you actually do need to modify. In that case, I'd encourage you to talk to someone you care about and trust who has been telling you to modify this part of your life. Invite them to share their point of view with you and fully listen to them. Once you've listened all the way through, if you still disagree with what they're saying, ask if you can share your hesitations or concerns and then invite them to address those disagreements. Again, listen fully. I've found that this process of inviting in a new point of view from someone close to you is the best and most high-probability approach to "unsticking" your previous point of view.

However, if you believe that you have truly revised your self-awareness in this area, it may be that the particular modifications you've chosen aren't working for you. In that case, I'd encourage you to look for other ways to make the change easier or more doable, other positive outcomes that are more meaningful to you, and other approaches to making the modification more normal and less weird. Remember, the goal here is to modify gracefully, elegantly, beautifully, and simply. And that's different for every person. Your modifications need to feel graceful *to you*.

Non-physical modifications

Before we leave this topic, I want to touch on the kind of modification that tends to be the most difficult for many of us. All the examples I've given in this chapter centered on physical changes: modifying your style, your exercise routine, your sex life, where you live. Even though modifying in those areas can be challenging, it's made somewhat easier because you're responding to tangible changes. If you can't walk without an assistive device or you can't get an erection, those things are hard to deny.

But what about when you need to make modifications based on changes in your mental capacity? I'm not even talking about dementia (although that's also an issue for millions of older people and can require heartbreaking modifications); I'm just talking about the decreases in focus, attention span, and memory that affect most seniors to some degree. Those changes can be tremendously difficult to acknowledge and respond to appropriately.

A powerful recent example was Joe Biden's decision, in July of 2024, to drop out of the US presidential race and not seek re-election, even though he was assured the Democratic nomination. After a very disappointing showing in the presidential debate the previous month, and upon consultation with many in his closest circle, he concluded that he would not be able to fulfill the duties of the president well for another four-year term—and that his clear diminution of abilities was likely to result in his losing the election.

Imagine how difficult that decision must have been! I'm sure Biden felt just as committed to his vision of America as he ever had and just as proud of what he and his team had accomplished over the previous three-and-a-half years. He probably even felt just as capable as ever, but that self-awareness wasn't accurate, and he somehow came to acknowledge that.

In addition to shifting his own self-concept, he would have had to overcome the stigma that exists regarding even mild cognitive decline in older people. Dozens of articles and studies have shown that most older people feel a good deal of shame and stress in thinking that their mental capabilities are diminishing, and that caregivers and society in general stigmatize a diminution in mental capability, leading to "discounting, discrediting, and dehumanizing."[5]

No wonder it can be hard for us to acknowledge when the mental requirements of a job are too much for us or when we need to step back from a leadership role or other mentally challenging endeavor we've loved.

I've had to deal with this issue myself. I decided in 2023 that I no longer wanted to sell or deliver services to clients; I had to acknowledge that the level of sustained physical and mental effort required for that would take a toll on me that I was not willing to pay. That was how I shifted my self-talk from where it started: *I can still contribute in this way and it's good for the company*, to my "modify gracefully" self-talk of: *There are other ways I can contribute that aren't so exhausting and that won't compromise my health and happiness*. I then ate my own caviar (more appealing than dog food, don't you think?) and figured out how to make that modification in a way that was easy, rewarding and normal.

I made it easier by creating a detailed and realistic plan with my partners to transfer my clients to them and other sellers in the company and by making videos to share with other deliverers and sellers some of what I've learned about working with clients. I made it more rewarding by using the time I reclaimed in ways that benefit the company (writing content, continuing my podcast, advising the senior team), benefit me (more time to explore and learn about my new Spanish culture and language), and benefit the world (writing this book, among other things). I've normalized it by figuring out how to talk to clients about the shift in a natural and positive way and by talking with others who are in this phase of life and have modified their work lives. I've also normalized it by shifting my own self-talk to acknowledge my decreased stamina and slightly slower pace of thinking as normal and acceptable–vs. scary or negative.

So, if you think you may need to make some non-physical modifications, I'd encourage you to use the same process we've worked through in this chapter–with the added encouragement to be especially kind to yourself in this transition and to take the time you need. I think history will see Joe Biden's decision as a very positive and valiant thing, and I suspect any decision you make in this realm will be both brave and supportive of your envisioned later life.

> **THE BIG IDEA: Later life requires a continual series of modifications. Making them intentionally and gracefully allows you the greatest degree of control, joy and satisfaction.**

---

[1] Hughes, J. M., Brown, R. T., Fanning, J., Raj, M., Bisson, A. N., Ghneim, M., & Kritchevsky, S. B. (2023). Achieving and sustaining behavior change for older adults: a Research Centers Collaborative Network workshop report. *The Gerontologist*, *63*(8), 1268-1278. https://www.ncbi.nlm.nih.gov/pmc/articles/PMC10474593/

[2] Kakara, R. (2023). Nonfatal and fatal falls among adults aged≥ 65 years—United States, 2020–2021. *MMWR. Morbidity and Mortality Weekly Report*, *72*. DOI: 10.15585/mmwr.mm7235a1

[3] Donizzetti, A. R. (2019). Ageism in an aging society: The role of knowledge, anxiety about aging, and stereotypes in young people and adults. *International journal of environmental research and public health*, *16*(8), 1329. doi: 10.3390/ijerph16081329.

[4] Flesia, L., Monaro, M., Jannini, E. A., & Limoncin, E. (2023, February). "I'm too old for that": the role of ageism and sexual dysfunctional beliefs in sexual health in a sample of heterosexual and LGB older adults: a pilot study. In *Healthcare* (Vol. 11, No. 4, p. 459). MDPI. https://www.mdpi.com/2227-9032/11/4/459

[5] Warren, A. (2023). The relationship between perceived stigma and perceived stress in cognitive decline: a survey of persons with mild cognitive impairment and their caregivers. *Frontiers in Psychology*, *14*, 1293284. https://www.ncbi.nlm.nih.gov/pmc/articles/PMC10740212/

12. Discover and Explore—Anything

"There is nothing more notable in Socrates than that
he found time, when he was an old man, to learn
music and dancing, and thought it time well spent."
—Michel de Montaigne

S ome of the most impressive and innovative inventions and works of art in human history have been created by people in the last third of their lives. Michelangelo designed the dome of the basilica of St. Peter's in Rome between the ages of 72 and 88. Stradivarius created his two most famous violins in his 90s. Mary Baker Eddy established the Christian Science Monitor when she was 87.

We used to think that such later-life creativity and learning was unusual; until recently, scientists assumed that our brain's ability to create new connections and acquire new learning diminished gradually and then stopped in midlife. However, recent research has shown that the opposite is true: new brain cells continue to emerge and develop well into old age. In fact, "neuroplasticity," the brain's ability to adapt and respond when confronted with new situations and input, is available throughout our lives.[1]

And what's the best way to maintain and enhance our brain's plasticity? By learning. Keeping our brains strong and active is definitely a use-it-or-lose-it proposition.

In addition to our brains being ready and willing to learn new things in this part of our lives, we also have additional advantages as later-in-life learners. First, as I've noted previously, most of us aren't raising kids or managing demanding careers in this part of our lives; we have more time to learn new things.

Second, due to the absence of said demanding careers which required us to focus our learning on things that would help us to get ahead, we have choice: we can learn anything we damn well please. We can decide to learn and practice things we might have longed to explore in our earlier lives but didn't have the time or bandwidth. For many people, the idea of learning something "just for fun" may be brand new—and once we get our heads around that possibility, it can be really motivating (we'll talk more about that later).

Finally, as one of the benefits of the digital age, we have many, many more resources available to us for learning new skills and acquiring new knowledge than existed even a decade ago. We can take online courses, find co-learner friends all over the world, and discover obscure texts and tutorials that would have been difficult or impossible to unearth previously.

Big Benefits of Learning…

In addition to all these factors that make it easier for us to acquire new skills and knowledge, it turns out there are a whole variety of added benefits in learning new things as older adults. A fascinating study was done recently with a group of adults between 58 and 86 years of age.[2] It was very simple: for three months, the study participants chose to study a new (to them) topic, taking three 2-hour classes a week. Course options included singing, drawing, iPad use, photography, Spanish, and music composition. At the end of the three-month study, each participant's memory and cognition had improved significantly. Even more interesting, when checked a year later, their cognitive abilities had improved even more—becoming similar to those of people 50 years younger. Sounds like the use-it-or-lose-it principle on steroids, from just a simple 3-month course of learning.

Other studies have shown that later-life learning is not only good for our brains, but also for our mental and physical health. Acquiring new skills and knowledge in later life can boost our mood, increase our self-esteem, improve social connections, lower our stress, and even improve our physical well-being.[3]

So, what gets in our way?

You may be nodding your head, thinking, *Yup, that's all true, but...I'm not really doing it.*

If learning new things in later life is so marvelous, why don't we do it more? And why is our self-talk about our lack of learning effort often so unsupportive? For example, you might be thinking to yourself, *I'm just too lazy,* OR *I'm too old and set in my ways to learn X,* OR *If I try to learn Y, I'll be surrounded by 25-year-olds, and they'll think I look dumb...*

When you stop to listen to your self-talk on this topic, you may be surprised at how negative you're being. But remember, learning new things is also a form of change, and we can have all the resistance and negativity (Difficult! Costly! Weird!) about learning that we have about any change.

So, as usual, let's start by revising any core negative self-talk you might be having about acquiring new skills or knowledge. Think of it as clearing away your mental underbrush so you have a clear field for learning.

Let's say you are having negative self-talk about learning new things. What's something hopeful and believable you could say to yourself instead as we start discussing what you might learn as part of your optimal later life?

One newly retired friend (who noticed that though he said he wanted to learn new things, wasn't doing it), tried this activity, and here's what he came up with: he recognized that he was saying to himself, *It's too much trouble to learn new things, I just want to laze around for the first time in my life.* He changed it to, *Lazing around is great fun–AND I also really want to explore some things I've never had a chance to look into before.* He told me that after he made the effort to revise his self-talk, he had signed up for a class on Roman history at a local college and was looking forward to it.

TRY IT

> My most negative self-talk about my ability/willingness to learn new things as an older adult:
>
>
>
>
>
> What do I want to say to myself instead?

How To Learn Like a Master

So, now that you're shifting your thinking to be more supportive of new learning, I want to offer you an approach to learning new things that I think you'll find helpful. I've already mentioned a previous book, *Be Bad First*,[4] in which I describe and explain four mental skills used throughout history by master learners. We call it the ANEW model:

Aspiration
Neutral Self-Awareness
Endless Curiosity
Willingness to Be Bad First

You may remember that we've already discussed the first two skills, Aspiration and Neutral Self-Awareness. Since you're somewhat familiar with them, we'll just touch on them lightly here to help you apply them in this context. Then I'll go into depth on Endless Curiosity and Willingness to Be Bad First, so you can take advantage of these key mental skills to help you learn whatever you'd like as a part of creating your best later life.

Aspiration

In Chapter 7, where I introduced the concept and the skill of managing your self-talk, I defined "aspiration" as "the motivation to learn or to do something differently or better." I also noted that learning something new requires a fairly high level of aspiration because new learning generally requires you to change your behavior—in other words, you *really* have to want to learn something new to actually do it.

We also talked about how to increase your level of aspiration so that you can follow through on your intentions and do those things (like managing your self-talk) that you know will benefit you but that you're not yet motivated enough to do. (If you want to refresh your memory about how this works, you're welcome to re-read the sections of Chapter 7 and Chapter 9 where we talked about how to increase your aspiration.)

But as you begin to think about which new things you might want to learn, let's make it easier for you: let's start with something that you believe you're highly motivated to learn—an area where you already have high aspiration.

How do you know you're highly motivated to learn something? Generally, when you think about it, you focus on all the benefits of learning that thing, and you think about the future where you're reaping those benefits. When we don't really want to learn something, on the other hand—when our aspiration is low—we tend to focus on all the ways in which it will be hard to learn (the anti-benefits, if you will), and we rarely think about the successful future where we've learned it.

So, what's some current topic or skill you're considering exploring that, when you think about it, you get excited imagining the rewards of knowing or doing it and you envision yourself experiencing those rewards?

It could be anything—any skill or area of knowledge. For example, when we first started spending more time in Spain a few years ago, I thought about how great it would be to be able to do anything I wanted to do in Spanish and how much easier and more fun it would make our time here. I also got excited (OK, I'm a nerd) about really understanding a second language the way I understand English. Those were the benefits of learning that appealed most to me.

Then I started imagining the future in which I was reaping those benefits: being able to make Spanish friends and have long conversations with them; taking courses in Spanish about the culture and history of this part of Spain; reading books in Spanish and enjoying and appreciating the writing; doing all my day-to-day tasks in Spanish easily and without problems.

Focusing on those benefits and envisioning that future worked for me: I've made the effort to learn and am mostly experiencing that future I envisioned. One small example: I'm now taking a class at the People's University here in Oviedo, "Mitos y Leyendas de Asturias y Oviedo" (Myths and Legends of Asturias and Oviedo), and it's really fun and interesting.

TRY IT

What's something I'd really like to learn?

How will learning this skill or area of knowledge benefit me?

What will the future look like when I'm reaping the benefits of my new learning?

As always, this is a very practical approach. If you do this activity but find, after a few weeks, that you're still not making the effort to start learning whatever topic you've chosen, it probably means you don't really aspire to learn it at this point. (NOTE: Another indication that your aspiration is low would be that even after you've noted possible benefits above, you find you're still thinking more about the obstacles and difficulties involved in learning this subject or skill.)

If this happens, just go back to the drawing board. Think of something else you'd really like to learn, and then, as above, note the benefits and envision your successful future where you're reaping the benefits of having learned it. (If you'd like more information about the possible benefits of learning something "just for fun," there are various studies that have shown all the myriad physical and emotional benefits of engaging in leisure activities.[5])

You can also draw on your vision. What's something that, if you learned it, would really support you in being the person you've said you want to be or in having the life you want to have?

And finally, if you want to make this first practice of using the ANEW model even easier, pick a subject that you've already taken some initial steps toward learning, as that's the best indication that your aspiration is high!

Neutral Self-Awareness

I introduced you to the idea of neutral self-awareness in the previous chapter, Modifying Gracefully, when we discussed how to know when you need to modify some aspect of your life. As you may remember, our self-awareness lives primarily in how we talk to ourselves about ourselves. We often don't see ourselves clearly, as reflected in our inaccurate (and often quite judgmental) interior monologue about ourselves. For instance, we might think to ourselves, *I have no ear for language; it will be impossible for me to learn a new one*, when that's simply not true. Or we might go in the opposite direction and say to ourselves, *I'm fantastic at learning languages, I'll be fluent in a few months!* Which is also probably not true.

It turns out that the very best and most useful place to start, when you're trying to learn anything, is reality. The more accurate and objective you can be about your starting point, the more likely it is that you will be able to find and access the right level of learning resources and have realistic expectations about your progress and outcomes.

Starting with a neutral and realistic interior monologue about yourself as a learner also means you'll be putting up fewer unnecessary and unhelpful obstacles to your learning. For example, if instead of saying to yourself, *I have no ear for language; it will be impossible for me to learn a new one,* you revise your self-talk to, *I've never really had success learning a new language, so I don't know which approach will work best for me,* that's a much more helpful (and neutral) starting frame.

So, what's the best way to become more neutrally self-aware? In the last chapter, we talked about the skill of becoming a "fair witness" of yourself in terms of whether you might need to modify some area of your life—and the same approach works well in assessing yourself as a learner:

- **Recognize/record your self-talk about where you are now in the area where you want to learn.**
- **Then ask yourself, "Is my self-talk accurate?"**
- **Where you're unsure, ask, "What facts do I have about myself in this area?"**
- **Revise your self-talk to be more accurate based on your answers.**

Let's apply this to the topic or skill you've decided you want to learn.

TRY IT

I intend to learn the following (topic or skill):

What am I saying to myself about my level of ability or expertise or my ability to learn in this area?

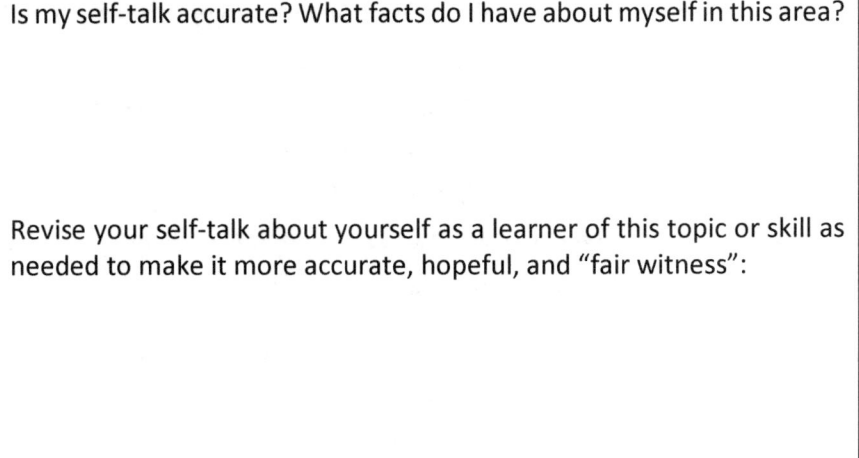

Is my self-talk accurate? What facts do I have about myself in this area?

Revise your self-talk about yourself as a learner of this topic or skill as needed to make it more accurate, hopeful, and "fair witness":

There's one other aspect of becoming neutrally self-aware as a learner that's important to mention here. As we've discussed, sometimes it's very difficult to see ourselves clearly. Partly, that's a result of the inevitable filters and blinders we tend to have when thinking about or reflecting on ourselves. Because we're so emotionally attached to ourselves and our abilities, and because our emotional history with ourselves is complex, including all the inputs from other people and the media telling us we're OK or not OK throughout our lives, it can sometimes be very hard to answer the question, "Is my self-talk about myself in this area accurate?"

So, I would strongly encourage you to think of a few people you can call upon in your life, people who see you clearly, want the best for you, and will tell you the truth. If you have folks in your life who fulfill all three of these criteria, they are a treasure; cherish them. Most of us have lots of people who fulfill one or even two of these: they want the best for us, or they're willing to be drop-dead honest with us. But all three is the trifecta: when someone truly has our best interests at heart and can see us accurately, and then is willing to tell us what they see, with love but also with honesty—that's rare. Those people will be especially helpful in any endeavor that requires you to be a fair witness to your circumstances and abilities as you embark upon something new.

For example, my husband wants nothing but the best for me and is willing and able to be honest—but he doesn't really see me clearly: he thinks I'm much better in most ways than I really am. It's a lovely quality to have in a life partner, but he's not a great fair witness for me. My son also has my best interests at heart and is more than willing to be honest, but he, unlike my husband, sees me with near-chilling clarity. It's sometimes hard to hear, but it's extraordinarily helpful.

Who's someone in your life you can call upon when you need some support for your fair witnessing? Note who they are and how you might request their support for your learning endeavors.

OK. So, whatever this area is where you've decided to learn, I hope your aspiration is now high, as witnessed by the fact that you're looking forward to the future where you know or can do the thing and you're starting to take steps to learn. You feel confident that you have a fairly accurate assessment of where you're starting from as a learner in this area, and your self-talk is neutral and supportive.

Now I want to share with you the two other powerful skills of master learners that will support you through your learning process in this or any other topic...especially when the going gets rough!

Endless Curiosity

I've become convinced over the years that true curiosity turbo-charges learning. So, what do I mean by "true curiosity"? I would define curiosity as a deep and abiding urge to understand and master new areas of knowledge or skill. That kind of curiosity is wired into us, and it drives much of the astonishing volume of learning that each of us does in our first few years. There's a wonderful book called *Brain Rules* by John Medina, where he talks about this phenomenon:

> "Let's look under the hood of an infant's mind, at the engine that drives its thinking processes and the motivating fuel that keeps its intellect running. This fuel consists of a clear, high-octane, unquenchable *need to know*[italics mine]. Babies are born with a deep desire to understand the world around them and an incessant curiosity that compels them to aggressively explore it. This need for explanation is so powerfully stitched into their experience that some scientists describe it as a drive, just as hunger and thirst and sex are drives.[6]"

This explains how we can go from being cute blobs at birth to being able to walk, talk, eat, play, and manipulate objects (and our parents) by the time we're three or four.

Unfortunately, that deep and endless curiosity that's intrinsic to us when we're born often gets socialized out of us as we age. Most of us learn, as teenagers, that it's better not to demonstrate too much curiosity—our friends think it's uncool, and the grown-ups around us often find it irritating. And by the time we're grown-ups, we often worry that being too curious at work will make us look dumb or naïve.

The good news is, we can re-engage that childhood curiosity; it's in there, lying fallow, waiting to be called upon. The learning we do as older adults is the perfect place to rediscover and use our "drive to know and understand."

If you feel like you've already re-found (or perhaps never lost) your curiosity—you're very, very lucky, and I suspect you're using it daily to explore the world, find out new things, and figure out how to be old in the best way possible.

But let's say that, like most of us, you've lost touch with your childhood curiosity along the way.

How Do We Get It Back?

If you'll forgive me an analogy, think of your curiosity as a fire that burned really brightly when you were a baby, and you needed it every day to figure out how to operate in the world. Then it probably died down, helped along by society's expectations and the demands of daily life. But I've found that, for almost everyone, the fire of curiosity hasn't gone out completely and can be re-stoked. Here's how it works:

To re-become endlessly curious:

- **Find your own curiosity "sparks"**
- **Fan the flames with self-talk and action**
- **Feed the fire of curiosity daily**

Find your own curiosity sparks. Even if you feel like you're not very curious right now, almost everyone has things (or even one thing) in their life about which they are truly curious. Those are the places to look for your un-extinguished sparks of curiosity. If you already have a hobby or hobbies, that's a great place to start looking for those sparks. Much-loved hobbies are the perfect medium for the expression of curiosity: endeavors that we enjoy so much that we spend time and energy exploring them even though we're not getting paid to do it, and where we don't worry (as much) about whether others will "think we're dumb" if we demonstrate our lack of knowledge. When it comes to our hobbies, we are curious. We want to know more, understand more deeply, get better, and discover how and why things work. And once you notice your own 'curiosity sparks,' you can transfer those sparks to other areas of learning (we'll talk about how to do that in just a bit).

Fan the flames with self-talk and action. This aspect of reclaiming your childhood curiosity relies first on a skill we've already been exploring: recognizing and managing your self-talk. It involves replacing any anti-curious self-talk you may have about learning with self-talk that supports your curiosity. Then, we'll talk about how that kind of self-talk naturally leads to action designed to satisfy your curiosity. In other words, curious self-talk supports taking practical steps to learn.

Feed the fire of curiosity daily. In this final part of re-engaging your childhood need-to-know, you make curiosity something you can draw on every day. Making curiosity a daily habit opens you up, makes you resilient and hopeful, sends you toward the new rather than away from it. It's the ideal foundation for learning (and, in fact, for doing all the things we've talked about throughout this book).

Find Your Curiosity Sparks

As I said, we often lavish our most ardent curiosity on our hobbies. For instance, a woman whose hobby is salsa dancing might take classes at night; participate in competitions; read books about the history of salsa; watch YouTube videos of world-class dancers; and talk to people who are highly skilled to learn how they practice and what they've done to overcome obstacles to improvement. In other words, she would explore salsa dancing in as many ways as are available to her, in order to *understand and master*; she is deeply curious about it.

TRY IT

Think about areas where those sparks of curiosity may still be burning in your own life. You can draw upon what you're already doing in those areas to ignite your curiosity in other areas. That is, by observing what you say to yourself and how you act when you're feeling curious, you can begin to create those same thoughts and actions in other areas where you want to get more curious. Let's give it a shot.

What's a topic about which you're already curious? (NOTE: If you're demonstrating some of the behaviors I noted above around a topic, you're curious about it.)

Reflect on the time you spend exploring this topic: What does that feel like? (For example: exciting, fun, invigorating, challenging, or satisfying.)

What's some of your self-talk about this topic? (For example: "How does that work?" or "I wonder if I could do that?" or "Why does that happen?")

Finally, what do you find yourself doing in response to your curious self-talk? (For example: reading more, asking more questions, trying some new things, finding a teacher, joining an affinity group.)

There you have it. Now that you know what your own curiosity looks and feels like, you can begin to transfer those "sparks" to new areas of learning. Let's go there....

Fan the Flames of Self-Talk and Action

Bringing your self-talk to your conscious awareness, as we've done several times over the past few chapters, allows you to sort the wheat from the chaff: to recognize and retain the self-talk that serves and supports you, and discard or re-think the rest.

That's what I'm encouraging you to do with the "self-talk of curiosity." When you reflected, in the exercise above, on your self-talk about a topic where you're already curious, you may have surfaced thoughts like:

> *How does that work?*
> *I wonder if I could do that?*
> *Why does that happen?*
> *How can I find out more?*
> *Why isn't that like this?*
> *I wonder what would happen if I tried this?*

You may notice a pattern here: I realized in observing good learners over the years, and working on my own skills as a learner, that curious self-talk most often begins with *Why...?*, *How...?*, or *I wonder...?* The need to understand and master is almost always the driving impulse behind those three sentence starters.

In my work at Proteus, over the years, I also noticed (in myself and our clients) what we came to call "anti-curiosity self-talk." That tends to sound like:

> *That's boring.*
> *Who cares?*
> *I already knew that.*
> *That doesn't matter.*
> *That's silly/dumb/too complicated.*
> *Whatever, dude.*

The pattern here, as you may notice, is *disinterest and dismissal*. And you might have already guessed that your first task in the "fanning the flames" part of re-igniting your curiosity is to shift your self-talk from anti-curious to curious in the areas where you want to learn.

The newly retired friend that I mentioned previously, who noticed that his overall unhelpful self-talk about learning was *I just want to laze around for the first time in my life*, also noticed that he had some specifically anti-curious self-talk about learning. When his wife brought up topics that she thought they might explore together, he found he was generally being negative and dismissive in response to her—and he realized that response arose from his interior monologue, which consisted of anti-curious phrases like, *That sounds boring*, and *I couldn't care less*.

When he did the previous exercise of "finding his curiosity sparks," he realized that he'd always been interested in ancient Western history, especially the Romans and Greeks. He noticed that he often had curious self-talk when thinking about it, like, *Why did the Romans put so much energy into expanding their Empire? How did the people whose lands they conquered relate to the Romans? I wonder how Greek society was different from Roman society?*

So, he did two things with this understanding. First, he focused on making his self-talk less anti-curious when his wife suggested an activity or area of knowledge, and second, he followed up on his existing curiosity by (as I noted previously) signing up for a course in Roman History at his local college.

With this example before you, let's take a shot at getting more curious about the topic you want to learn.

TRY IT

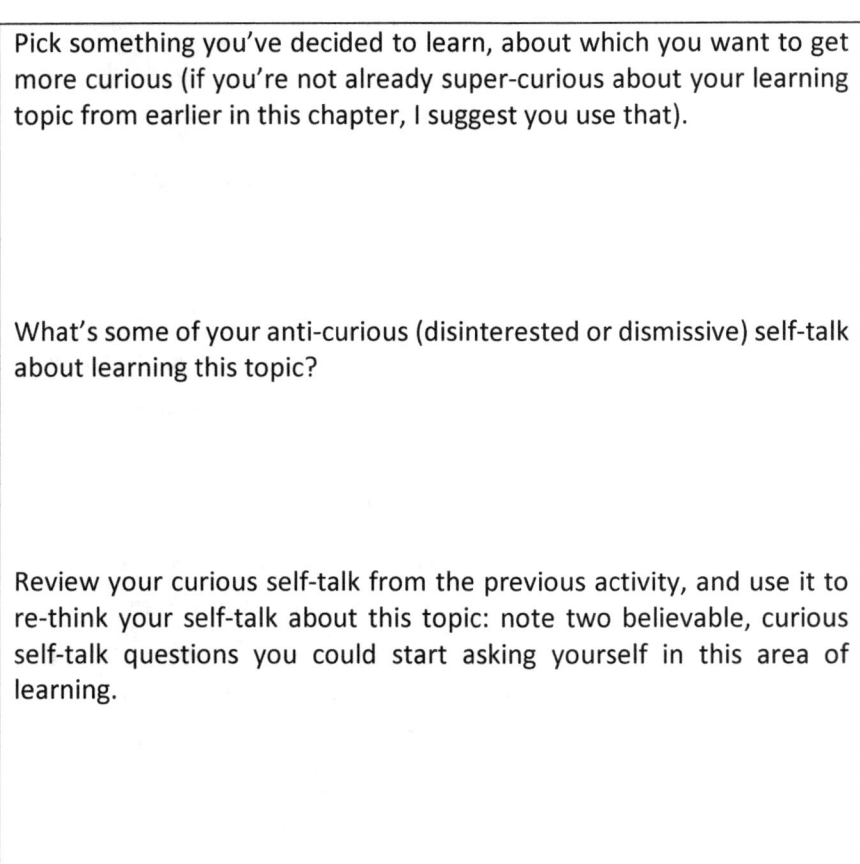

Pick something you've decided to learn, about which you want to get more curious (if you're not already super-curious about your learning topic from earlier in this chapter, I suggest you use that).

What's some of your anti-curious (disinterested or dismissive) self-talk about learning this topic?

Review your curious self-talk from the previous activity, and use it to re-think your self-talk about this topic: note two believable, curious self-talk questions you could start asking yourself in this area of learning.

Congratulations—you've just transferred your spark of curiosity from one area to another. Now, let's help it burn brighter.

Following Self-Talk with Action

When you're genuinely curious about something, the "How," "Why," and "I wonder" questions you're asking yourself demand answers, and you'll automatically take action to find those answers: that's how real learning happens.

Recently, I decided I wanted to learn how to crochet. I already do a lot of knitting, and one of my grandkids sent me a picture of a blanket she would like to have me make for her. Looking at it, I realized it was a crochet pattern. I ultimately figured out how to knit something very similar instead, but the experience made me want to learn to crochet. I made sure my aspiration was sufficient, and I got clear about where I was starting from. Then, I worked on getting curious.

I wonder if I could learn this from YouTube? I thought to myself–and followed that curious self-talk by opening my computer, going to YouTube and searching for "learning to crochet." It seemed simple and doable, so then I found myself asking another curiosity-based question, *I wonder if there's somewhere to get crochet supplies near here?* The action that followed was simple reflection, followed by the ah-ha that a general store right next to our local supermarket almost certainly has crochet hooks. So, next time I go to the store, I'll pick up a crochet hook, pop open my computer, and I'll be on my way.

You may have noticed that the actions that followed my curious self-talk were simple efforts designed to answer the questions raised. It's a natural progression: first, you think *How...?*, or *Why...?*, or *I wonder...?* and then you want to answer the question. We're built to follow that progression: it's how we've made every human advance in skill or knowledge from figuring out how to make fire to the latest discoveries in gene therapy. The main thing that gets in the way of that progression from curious self-talk to curious action is a resurgence of anti-curious self-talk. For example, if the crocheting video on YouTube initially looked too complicated, my self-talk response could have been, *This is silly. I've got more important things to think about.* Classic disinterest and dismissal, which would have immediately squelched my impulse to get a crochet hook and try out what I was seeing on YouTube.

Recall the self-talk model of *recognize*, *record*, *re-think* and *repeat*: this is the point in re-engaging your curiosity where the "repeat" step is going to come in very handy. As adults, most of us have learned to talk ourselves out of following up on our curiosity. And it tends to be even more true as we age and can get more set in our ways. You feel curious about something, and instead of doing something to satisfy that curiosity, you tell yourself it's not important, or that you're fine the way you are, or that you'll look dumb—you've reverted to unhelpful, curiosity-killing self-talk.

When this happens, there are two simple things you can do to set yourself back on the path of curiosity and learning. First, simply go back to your original curious self-talk. In my case, that would have meant saying to myself, *No, I really do want to see if I can learn this*. (It's quite liberating to realize that you can "talk back" to your own unhelpful self-talk, that you don't have to believe the unsupportive things your inner voice tells you.)

Second, choose follow-up actions that are easy *for you*. For example, in my case, I'm constantly on the internet, looking for answers to questions or finding out how to do things—so that's always an easy first action for me to take to follow my curiosity. For someone else, asking a friend might be an easier and more natural first action. And for another person, just trying something out might be the easiest thing to do first.

Now that you've got some tools for turning your newly minted curious self-talk into action, let's put them to use.

TRY IT

Review your new-made curious self-talk from the last activity, and note 1 or 2 simple (for you) actions you'll take to answer the questions you've raised:

1.

2.

If anti-curious self-talk arises that could keep you from taking those actions, how will you repeat your curious self-talk to allow yourself to keep learning?

Feed the Fire of Curiosity Daily

If you start applying the tools we've been talking about—shifting your self-talk from anti-curious to curious and taking action to pursue your curiosity—you'll find a powerful shift beginning to occur inside you. The momentum toward being largely incurious, which for most of us increases throughout our lives, will slow and begin to reverse. More and more often, you'll be sitting in your living room, taking a walk, or reading a book and find yourself thinking, *Huh. I wonder if...?* or *Why does that...?* or *How can I...?* That's your natural curiosity re-awakening, re-igniting.

I'm assuming, since you've read this far, that you want that to happen; that you're seeing your curiosity as an asset, and you want to unleash it even further in order to support you in creating the later life you most want. If so, there's one simple thing you can do to turbo-charge your curiosity: Create your own personal "curiosity match" and use it every day.

You know how a physical match works: it's the simplest and most reliable way to start a fire. A curiosity match is a piece of self-talk that works for you to simply and reliably spark your curiosity. Once you've identified your own curiosity match, you can apply it whenever and wherever you like.

Michelangelo, one of the greatest master learners in Western history, had a curiosity match. It was *I am still learning–Ancora Imparo* in Italian. His biographers tell us that he said it often: as a response to compliments; when approaching a new problem; in asking others for their knowledge or insight. What a wonderful spark for curiosity! My own curiosity match is, *I'd love to find out more about that*. That works for me: it's accurate (I mostly *do* want to find out more about things), it encourages me to get as curious as I'd like, and it leads directly to great curiosity-based self-talk and action.

Like all good self-talk, your curiosity match has to be something that's true for you. And it has to be something that will support further curiosity. The easiest way to craft a curiosity match for yourself is to notice something positive you're already saying to yourself about being curious and apply it more broadly. Before we leave this ANEW skill, let's build you a really good match that will help re-ignite your Endless Curiosity daily.

TRY IT

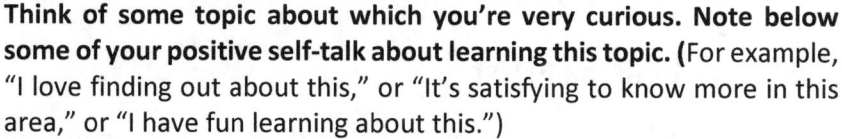

Think of some topic about which you're very curious. Note below some of your positive self-talk about learning this topic. (For example, "I love finding out about this," or "It's satisfying to know more in this area," or "I have fun learning about this.")

Choose one of your statements and revise it to apply more broadly. (For example, "I love finding out about things," or "It's satisfying to know more," or "I have fun learning.")

There you have it: a first draft of your very own, custom-built curiosity match. I encourage you to try it out over the next little while as you think about things you might want to learn.

If it doesn't work–if it doesn't spark your curiosity in these areas, then build another "match" and try that. You're a novice in this area of consciously developing your curiosity, and so it's inevitable that you won't be great at the beginning. Nobody starts out being an expert at things they haven't done before.

Even though that's true, and even though we all understand rationally that there's no possible way to be good at something you're just starting to learn, our discomfort with being novices is, nonetheless, nearly universal. That discomfort is the final barrier to becoming a world-class learner. Being willing to "look dumb"–to make mistakes, be clumsy, and not know—is the final frontier in becoming a master of mastery, and that's where we're going next.

Willingness to Be Bad First

Just as most little children are much better than most adults at being curious, they are also better at being novices. It's what they're used to, every moment of the day: the world is new to them, and they're figuring it out—they don't put the expectation on themselves that they have to be experts, to know everything already. At the same time, they believe that they'll be able to get better (at least those who have been raised in reasonably loving, non-punitive households) because their entire life to date has been an unbroken string of getting better at things. Here's a kid's world: "I didn't know how to talk; now I do. I didn't know how to put on my clothes; now I do. I didn't know how to catch a ball, ride a bike, sing a song, cut with scissors, count to 20, close the door, say my colors—now I do."

Sadly, as adults, just as we often lose touch with our curiosity, we also lose that wonderful childlike ability to be OK with being novices. Unfortunately, that discomfort with being a beginner really gets in the way as we age. As I've mentioned, my husband and I have been putting a lot of effort into learning Spanish as an important part of our transition to living in northern Spain. It turns out that a lot of what makes language learning more difficult for older adults is not a brain problem, but rather an expectation problem. We don't like being beginners as older adults, and we assume that the fact that we're not already good at something at our advanced age means we're not going to be able to get good at it.[7]

In simple terms, as older adults, we have a hard time "being bad first," and that becomes the main impediment to our learning. So, let's talk about how to get better at being a novice in this stage of life.

To become willing to be bad first:

- **Fully accept being not-good**
- **Believe in your ability to get good**
- **"Bridge" from what you're already good at**

As you might have suspected, our willingness (or unwillingness) to be bad first lives mostly in the same place as our neutral self-awareness and endless curiosity: it's all about how you talk to yourself. So, let's take your skills in managing your self-talk and apply them to becoming great at being bad.

Fully accept not-good. When we're trying to learn something new, especially in front of others, and we make inevitable mistakes, our self-talk can go something like this: *Oh my god, I'm such a loser. This is awful. I hate it. I'm 70 years old, for god's sake, I'm not supposed to be bumbling around like this.* Not helpful, and deeply uncomfortable. We'll focus on transforming that unproductive self-talk in learning situations into accurate, believable self-talk based on the understanding that being bad at things you're doing for the first time is not only acceptable but inevitable.

Believe in your ability to get good. Once you're no longer resisting your initial "badness," you need to assert to yourself that you're capable of moving beyond that novice state, of getting good at whatever it is you're trying to learn. Fortunately, we all have a lifetime of getting better at things that we can reference to support this. You'll learn to balance your "acceptance of not-good" self-talk with "self-belief" self-talk, which will free you to solve the learning challenges before you.

Bridge from what you're already good at. With this more realistic and supportive self-talk in place, you'll be better able to access and use any related skills and knowledge, applying what you already know to what you're just beginning to learn.

Fully Accept Not-Good

If you stop and listen to what you're saying to yourself as you're trying to learn something new, you'll notice that the vast majority of it focuses on resisting and bad-mouthing (bad-minding?) yourself about your novice state. For example: *Aagh! I'm so clumsy/stupid/slow! Why can't I figure this out/do this right/get it together?* When we talk to ourselves like that, we feel embarrassed, helpless, silly, awkward, anxious–maybe even depressed or hopeless. And those feelings tend to lead to even worse, less helpful self-talk; the kind of insidious self-talk that predicts complete failure in our learning efforts. (*I'm such an idiot. Why do I even try? I'll never be able to learn this...or anything!*)

Shifting your resistant and self-castigating self-talk into the self-talk of acceptance can create an immediate positive shift in your emotions and a remarkable sense of mental clarity.

Whenever I'm trying to understand and develop a new way of approaching something, I always use myself as a guinea pig. And this skill, of willingness to be bad first, is almost always the hardest for me. When I first started trying to learn Spanish eight years ago, one of my first actions was to have simple conversations in Spanish with one of my Proteus colleagues who is fluent in Spanish as well as a number of other languages (I admit I'm still jealous). Before attempting these conversations with her, I had to work hard to change my self-talk to "accepting being not-good." I would consciously say, *I'm going to be bad at this for a while because I haven't done it before. That's just how it is.* Saying that to myself felt almost like setting down a physical weight. Just acknowledging and accepting the reality of my novice-ness made me feel immediately less pressured, more capable and hopeful.

And then something very exciting happened. Because I accepted that I simply wouldn't be good to start with, I behaved very differently.

Having decided I had nothing to prove to Vanessa or myself, I could just listen to her, try saying a few things myself, ask her for corrections or translations, and try it again. By the end of the first conversation, Vanessa said, "It seems like you're already improving. I thought this would be a lot harder for you; usually, people are so hard on themselves when they make mistakes!"

Exactly.

You've already been practicing the skill of managing your self-talk, so let's apply the "recognize, record, revise, repeat" model here. In preparation for my first (and subsequent) conversations with Vanessa, I **recognized** my "anti-being bad" self-talk about it, which was: *This is going to be frustrating and embarrassing. I hate not being able to do things. I hope I don't suck at this too much.* I **recorded** it by writing it down, and as I reviewed it, I tried to be as fair a witness as possible. I was able to **revise** my self-talk to be, as I noted above: *I'm going to be bad at this for a while because I haven't done it before. That's just how it is.* I prepared to **repeat** that self-talk whenever my "anti-novice" self-talk reared its ugly head.

TRY IT

Now it's your turn. Let's focus on the topic you've decided to learn.

What's some of your "anti-being bad" self-talk about this topic?

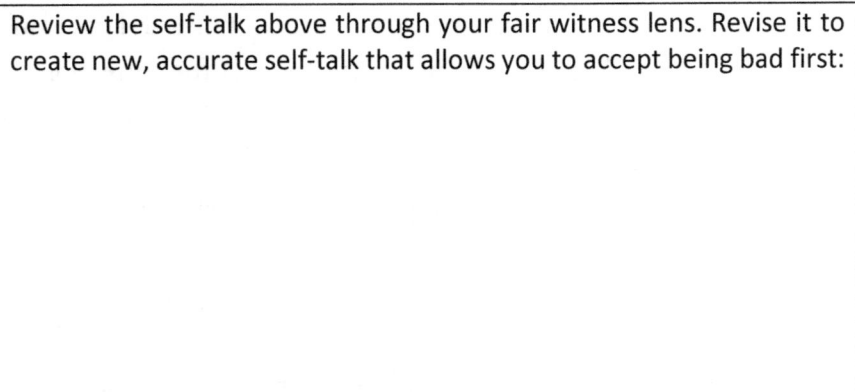

Review the self-talk above through your fair witness lens. Revise it to create new, accurate self-talk that allows you to accept being bad first:

If you're like most people, you'll definitely have to repeat this one—our negative self-talk about being bad at things is particularly sticky and insidious. I had to remind myself, *"I'm going to be bad at this for a while because I haven't done it before. That's just how it is,"* many times before, during, and after that conversation!

Believe in Your Ability to Get Good

Too often, even if we are able to shift our initial self-talk when learning to some form of accepting not-good, the self-talk that all too often tends to follow immediately is *And I'm going to be bad at it forever. I'll never get any better.* We've already talked about how we can be dreadfully (and unrealistically) hard on ourselves.

To explode those very pernicious beliefs about your lack of learning ability, you need only to look at your own life in a fair witness way. If you review your life objectively, you'll remember that you've gotten better at literally thousands of things. Think about what you were able to do when you were five years old; think of all the things you can do now. All human beings can learn and grow. Period. So, when that voice in your head starts to predict that not only will you be bad first, but that you'll *always* be bad—you can shift that self-talk to assert, completely accurately, that *I've gotten good at lots of things in my life. I'll be able to get better at this.*

You can then make your self-talk of self-belief even more powerful by acknowledging specific things that you've learned, or qualities in yourself that you know make you a particularly good learner. For instance, my balancing self-talk in approaching my first Spanish conversation was, *I'm sure I can learn this. I love language, and I'm good at getting curious and figuring out what's not working when I'm faced with something new.*

TRY IT

Now you get to create this second "balancing" self-talk statement to use in approaching your new learning.

Review the "accepting not-good" self-talk you created in the previous activity (if you like, you can note it again below).

Now create an accurate, simple self-talk statement that reflects your belief in your ability to get good in this area over time. (Acknowledge your history of learning similar skills or your strengths as a learner to make it even more personal and powerful.)

OK. What you've just built is a very powerful psychological tool to support your learning: you have a balanced self-talk statement that gives you permission to be a novice AND supports your ability to learn and get better over time. Congratulations! You can use this balanced self-talk whenever you need it: in learning the topic or skill that you've chosen in this chapter and in learning anything you want (or need) to explore in the service of creating your best later life.

Bridge From What You Already Know

One final support for being bad first as you learn new things. Since you've lived for a while and have learned a bunch of things, whenever you're learning something new, it's likely that you've done some related learning at some point. This is true even when the learning seems entirely new and different to you. For example, one of my interviewees for this book was offered a board position a few years ago with a non-profit focused on helping immigrants and their families settle in their new communities. She was surprised, since her professional background had been in marketing. But as she spoke to the board chairman, she realized that her expertise in messaging could help the organization better communicate with the communities involved, to help them understand the benefits the newly arrived residents might bring.

On the other hand, I've often seen people go too far in the other direction: assuming that new learning is *exactly* like what they already know. I once managed someone who unconsciously used this approach to hide her fear of being bad. For example, at one point (this was many years ago, when our business was quite small), we were planning to start using accounting software rather than doing our books manually on Excel spreadsheets. As we were reviewing a demo of the software, she said, somewhat dismissively, "Oh, this is just like what I've been doing." I looked at her, puzzled. "Really?" I responded. "It seems quite different to me." "No," she assured me, "it's pretty much the same."

Sadly, it took our accountant months to convince her that it was, indeed, different, so that she would be open to learning the new software to simplify and improve our financial approach.

In other words, using this tactic of "bridging" in the service of being bad first requires a kind of Goldilocks approach: not too little and not too much, but just right: you don't want to either under-estimate or over-estimate the relevance of previous learning when you're approaching a new area of skill or knowledge.

Your biggest ally in finding that sweet spot will be your curiosity. When thinking about learning something new, I encourage you to first ask yourself, *I wonder what skills or knowledge I have that are related to this new area of learning?* When something comes to mind as a possibility, you can ask yourself a second curious question: *How are my existing skills similar to and different from what will be required in this new learning area?*

I've found that if I ask myself (or encourage someone I'm working with to ask themselves) these two curiosity-based questions when entering into a new learning situation, they're much more likely to be able to figure out how to use their existing skills and knowledge to support their learning in the new area.

TRY IT

Let's apply this final tactic to your own be bad first challenge.

As you think about your learning topic (about which you now have supportive self-talk that balances accepting-not-good with self-belief), ask yourself: I wonder what skills or knowledge I already have that are related to this new topic?

Thinking of the skill or expertise you believe is most relevant, ask yourself: How is this similar to and different from what will be required in learning the new topic or skill?

Your Toolkit is Full

That's it. You now have the four powerful ANEW tools you need to acquire the new skills and knowledge you decide to learn to make your later life more enjoyable and engaging, and to better fulfill your later life vision. You've learned the basics of how to make yourself *aspire* to learn the things you want to learn. You know how to become more *neutrally self-aware,* more objective and accurate about your strengths and weaknesses as you approach new learning. You've learned some simple secrets for re-engaging your own *endless curiosity.* Now, you also know the most important skill for new learning: accepting and moving through the inevitable necessity of *being bad first.*

A Wonderful Example

As I age, I'm continually looking for inspiring and clear examples of people who are creating great later lives for themselves, especially those who are master learners. One of my favorite old-age role models—and someone who especially embodied the "discover and explore anything" approach—was a woman named Tao Porchon Lynch. At her death in 2020 at the age of 101, she was the oldest active yoga teacher in the world. In fact, she taught her last class a few days before she died. And though she had taught yoga for much of her adult life and had continued to learn and improve her craft throughout her career, it was by no means the only thing she learned as an older person.

Tao began to do ballroom tango dancing in her 70s, and in her 80s and 90s, she won hundreds of competitions in partnership with dancers 50 or 60 years her junior. In her 50s, she and her husband founded the American Wine Society, and in her 70s, she became the publisher and editor-in-chief of a wine appreciation magazine. She wrote and published her autobiography at the age of 95.

Porchon Lynch was also a fabulous example of the joy of learning and of using the ANEW skills—she was deeply curious and didn't mind being a novice, and until her final days, she would often say, "Don't let age dictate what you can and cannot do."

Another thing I noticed about Porchon Lynch as an example of later-life learning is that much of her learning and exploration happened in collaboration or in company with others. And connecting with others is the focus of our next chapter....

THE BIG IDEA: We have the time, bandwidth and capability to learn new things now—and it benefits us dramatically while supporting us in creating the life we most want.

---

[1] Rauchman, R. (2023). *Neuroplasticity and healthy aging: What you need to know.* Pacific Neuroscience Institute. https://www.pacificneuroscienceinstitute.org/blog/brain-health/neuroplasticity-and-healthy-aging-what-you-need-to-know/

[2] Wu, R., Church-Lang, J. (2023). *To stay sharp as you age, learn new skills.* Scientific American.https://www.scientificamerican.com/article/to-stay-sharp-as-you-age-learn-new-skills/

[3] Seasons Retirement Communities. (n.d.). *10 Amazing benefits of lifelong learning for older adults.* https://seasonsretirement.com/benefits-of-lifelong-learning/

[4] Andersen, E. (2016). Be bad first: Get good at things fast to stay ready for the future. Routledge

[5] Pressman, S. D., Matthews, K. A., Cohen, S., Martire, L. M., Scheier, M., Baum, A., & Schulz, R. (2009). Association of enjoyable leisure activities with psychological and physical well-being. *Biopsychosocial Science and Medicine, 71*(7), 725-732. https://www.ncbi.nlm.nih.gov/pmc/articles/PMC2863117/

[6] Medina, J. (2008). Brain Rules: 12 principles for surviving and thriving at work, home and school. Pear Press

[7] Singleton, D., & Záborská, D. (2020). Adults learning additional languages in their later years. *Journal of Multilingual Theories and Practices, 1*(1), 112-124.https://doi.org/10.1558/jmtp.15361

A Thread That Runs Through Everything...

13. Connection Is More Important Than Ever

*"Those who love deeply never grow old, they may die
of old age, but they die young."* —Benjamin Franklin

We are tribal creatures. From the moment we're born, much more helpless and dependent than any other mammalian species, we require support and interaction with our fellow humans to grow and flourish. Reams of historical, biological and anthropological research over the past few decades have reinforced our identity as fundamentally social creatures. It even turns out that one of the main reasons our brains are so relatively large in proportion to our bodies, compared with other animals, is that the social interaction so essential to our surviving and thriving is very cognitively demanding. Our brains have evolved to better support our ability to be social.[1]

And like the other things we need to survive as individuals and as a species–food, sleep, water, sex–we crave social connection when we don't get it.[2] The name for that craving is loneliness.

The Loneliness Epidemic

It may seem counterintuitive that anyone would be lonely in this loud, bustling, highly populated world. But as we all know, being surrounded by people doesn't mean feeling connected to them. In fact, many studies have shown that more people now feel lonelier than ever before and that loneliness is especially prevalent among older people–and is growing.[3].

Why is this? Many of the social connections that supported us in previous eras have frayed or disappeared. A hundred years ago, most older people lived with or near their families and were deeply connected with the day-to-day lives of their children and grandchildren, as well as more extended family bonds–nieces and nephews, cousins, in-laws. Older people were also deeply involved in their communities and their religious groups. These days, as society has become more mobile, older people are much more likely to live far away from their closest family members, and many of us are no longer connected to local religious or community organizations. In addition, people who are now over 60 are more likely to be childless than in any previous generation.

Retirement, or even semi-retirement, also erodes important social connections. At the end of 2023, I stopped selling and delivering to clients and now only spend about 10 hours a week working with my colleagues at Proteus–and it has made me understand how many of my connections were professional and how much of my social needs were being met through work. In fact, because my profession has been such a major part of my life for so many years, the relationships that arose at and through work happened without a lot of effort. I didn't really have to go looking for people I enjoyed spending time with and with whom I had a lot in common: they were right there. It seems this is true for lots of us who are now contemplating retirement–in fact, a recent survey shows that 61% of workers fear retiring more than death. And though some of people's concerns are financial, almost half (48%) of those surveyed were concerned about "feeling disconnected from society."[5]

And Closest to Home…

Our most intimate connections are dissolving as well: more older people are getting divorced these days than in any previous period. In 1990, only 9% of divorces occurred in couples over 50; in 2019, that older age group accounted for 36% of divorces…and the only age group where the rate of divorce is currently increasing is the over-65s. I've also experienced this statistic: My first marriage broke up when I was in my 50s, and it was hugely scary and disorienting. I'm deeply grateful that I met and married my husband Patrick, but that isn't the case for many late-in-life divorced people; only about half of divorced people over 65 remarry.[6]

And finally, the saddest and most inevitable breaker of social connections: death. Spouses, parents, friends and siblings die, leaving us bereft of our most important connections.

As a result of all these factors, more older adults are living alone than ever before. About 30% of people aged 65 and older in the US and Europe live alone (more women than men); sixty years ago, that number was 1 in 10.[7]. And while it's not inevitable that those living alone will be lonely, it's certainly more likely.

And loneliness doesn't just feel bad–it's bad for us in many other ways, too. Older adults who report being lonely also report feeling more stress and depression, have worse health profiles (including more cardiovascular disease), have worse cognition and memory, and are more likely to die at younger ages.[3]

So, if the current state of society makes it more likely that we will be socially under-connected as old people, and that's bad for our health as well as our psychological and emotional well-being, how do we re-connect?

It's a Change Problem

Having to make new connections and connect in new ways as older adults is (you won't be surprised to realize) a change. And, as we've been discussing for the last three chapters, change is hard.

The good news is that you now have an understanding of how to go through change successfully (particularly the change of learning new things) and some tools for doing so. And more good news: many of the other tools and approaches we've discussed here will also be helpful in making new human connections in this third act of your life. Let's dive in.

Start with your vision

When you created (or honed) your later life vision in Chapter 4–your simple expression of who you want to be and what you want your life to be like as you age–I'll bet you anything it contained social elements. If you look back at my vision elements and the examples I shared with you of other seniors with whom I've spoken and worked, you'll note that every one of them involves other people, either directly ("my goal is to enjoy my life by helping others make progress") or indirectly ("I am kinder, slower and smarter than I used to be"–you have to be kind *to* someone).

To get clearer about the social aspects of your own vision, I encourage you to reflect on the future you outlined for yourself and think about the kinds of connections you will want and need to have in order to achieve both aspects of your vision, for yourself and for your life. For example, I realized that to "discover, support and enjoy" other people, I needed friends–and friends who shared some of my interests.

Do you have those connections now? If so, great. If not, briefly note the connections your vision will require below.

TRY IT

What kinds of human connections will I need to achieve my later-life vision? (For example: friendships, mentor relationships, affinity groups, professional associations, family bonds)

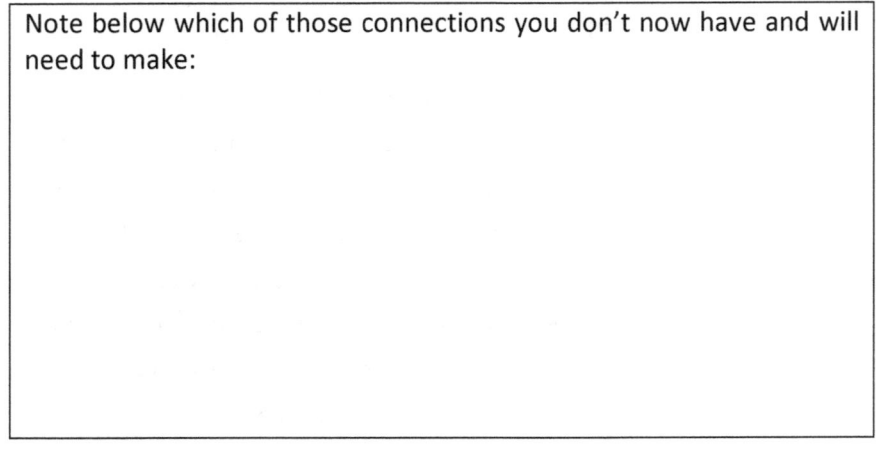

Note below which of those connections you don't now have and will need to make:

More About Community

I noted earlier that when I mostly retired last year, I was surprised to find that I was also largely disconnecting from my main source of friendship and social connectedness. Since I hadn't really had to focus on making friends for many years–and especially since I'm now mostly living in a new (to me) country–I felt a little overwhelmed about how to make new friends.

But I realized that the first thing I would have to do would be to get more intentional and proactive both about the kind of people I wanted to connect with and how to go about doing it. First, I took advantage of what I was already learning about "leading my crew," our topic in Chapter 6. I realized that many of the qualities I looked for in the people who would support my success as I aged were the same qualities I would want in friends. For example, you may remember that when we were looking for someone who could help us redesign our kitchen in Spain, I decided that I wanted people who were "highly collaborative, great listeners, curious, and extremely competent but also open and humble."

As I reflected on that, I realized that the only one I didn't care so much about in my friendships was "extremely competent"–but that a version of that, "very reliable," was indeed important to me. I also came to the conclusion that while a good sense of humor isn't so critical to me in working relationships, I really love having that in personal relationships.

So, the characteristics I was looking for in friends: Highly collaborative, great listener, curious, very reliable, open and humble, and with a good sense of humor. When I had gotten clear about that list, I vetted it against my best friends over the years (including my husband), and it turned out that the list had captured reality: my dearest friends have all or most of those characteristics.

This may seem like a strange approach; you've probably never done this before. Most of us make our friends fairly unconsciously through work or school, parents of our kids' friends, or people who share hobbies or habits with us. But as we've noted, a lot of these automatic social mechanisms don't work as well or aren't as easily available as we age.

I believe this more intentional approach to creating friendships as we age has another advantage, too. Because our approach to creating connections tends to be more haphazard early in life, the quality of those connections can vary wildly. My daughter-in-law, who is marvelous at connecting with people, realized a few years ago that while she had tons of "friends," too many of those relationships weren't nourishing and healthy–they weren't with the kinds of people she most wanted to be friends with as she became a parent and moved into middle age.

The quality of our friendships is even more important as we move into our third act: there's a now-famous phrase, "life's too short to deal with assholes," that becomes more and more true and accurate the older we get. If I only have 20 or 30 more years to live, I want to make sure I'm spending time with the kinds of people who support me to live my best life–and for whom I can do the same.

This clarity and intentionality is not only important in new friendships but in existing ones, as well. As I started to get clearer about the qualities

I most want in my new relationships, it made me value my deepest current relationships even more and inspired me to make sure that I am attending to and nourishing them. (In a little while, we'll talk more about how to strengthen existing relationships at the same time you're creating new ones.)

In that spirit, I invite you to look back at the qualities for your "crew" that you chose in Chapter 6 and modify them as needed to end with your most important friendship criteria.

TRY IT

My desired "crew" qualities from Chapter 6:

How would I modify those qualities to apply to new friends?

Managing Your Mindset

OK, now you have a sense of the types of human connections you'll need to support your vision and the kind of people with whom you'll most enjoy making those connections. Before we talk about how to find those people, let's look at how you're talking to yourself about this whole topic.

Now, you may be one of those folks for whom making friends is like breathing (I have a friend like that here in Spain, and she continually astonishes me with her natural friend-creation ability). But as I noted earlier, if you're like most people, the conscious making of friends may be a big change for you. And, like most externally-imposed changes, you may see it as difficult, costly and weird....and your self-talk most likely reflects that. When I realized last year that I was going to have to make the effort to make new friends in Spain if I wanted more social connection, I realized I was saying to myself, *This sucks. I don't know how to make friends, and it's even harder here where I don't speak the language very well. I'm going to feel like an idiot. I don't want to have to do this!* In other words, I was telling myself that it was going to be super-difficult, super-costly and super-weird.

Because I generally try to practice what I preach, I revised my self-talk about this challenge to make it more accurate, hopeful, and focused on how this change could be easy (or at least doable), rewarding and even normal. Here's what I came up with:

> *Well, I like people, and I'm getting clearer about the kinds of people I like being friends with. I'm sure I'll get better at making friends as I go. It may be awkward at times, but I think it will be worth it.*

It seems to be working for me; I'm making wonderful friends here in Spain. I encourage you to take a few minutes now to clean up your own self-talk about making connections.

TRY IT

Any current negative self-talk I'm having about the process of making new connections:

How I'll revise that self-talk to be more accurate and hopeful as I approach making new connections:

Getting Curious and Taking Action

OK. You're clear on the kinds of people you're looking for in your envisioned life, and you've reduced your own mental and emotional interference by managing your self-talk on this topic.

Now you get to find some great new people to connect with. Where to start?

We'll pull from what we discussed in the last chapter about learning new things: let's get curious. You may remember when we talked about the "self-talk of curiosity." When we want to find out more about something to get better at it and ultimately master it, we ask ourselves a lot of "How?" "Why?" and "I wonder?" questions. Not all curious questions start that way, but it's a great place to begin and will get your curiosity motor revving. As I started to think about making new connections in Spain, some of my curious questions were, *How do other expats make connections here? I wonder if there are activities I could do here that would attract like-minded people?* and *Why don't I find other people in the city who are looking for new international friends?*

And, as we noted in the last chapter, the beauty of curious self-talk is that it begs to be answered—it moves you to action. So, when I thought, *How do other expats make connections here?* I followed up on my curiosity by joining a Facebook group called "Expats in Asturias–International Community." I joined a sub-group of that group called "Ladies in Oviedo" (our city). Through that group, I met a wonderful woman named Coca, who has become one of my best friends here (and has all my favorite qualities). Meeting Coca was a double bonus because she's the aforementioned natural-friend-maker, and she has introduced me to others, including another woman, Julie, who has also become a lovely friend.

In response to my *I wonder if there are activities I could do here that would attract like-minded people?* question, I found and joined a yoga class—mostly because I wanted to make a habit of doing yoga as part of my overall vision, but also because I figured it might be a great place to make friends. And I have indeed made two wonderful friends, Marita and Carmen, both of whom are retired professors and delightful humans.

It's important to note that I also walked down a few dead-end paths: for instance, I tried going to an English/Spanish language meet-up in a local bar in response to my third question (*Why don't I find other people in the city looking for new international friends?*), and it was a complete bust—too loud, too transactional—and it included none of the kinds of people I wanted for friends. I mention this so your self-talk doesn't try to sabotage your efforts if one or more of them doesn't work out.

Now, you can play with this. I've noted the activity below (and like all the activities here, it's also at thenewoldbook.com), but I suggest that you stretch this one out and take it off the page. Think about it over the next few days and weeks. When you think of a curious question about how to make new connections that engages you and makes you want to take action—just do it. Of course, you can certainly write it down if you think it will help you remember or make you more likely to follow up, but the more important thing is simply to move forward and explore possible ways to connect. Think of this activity as a catalyst for you to start making new connections...

TRY IT

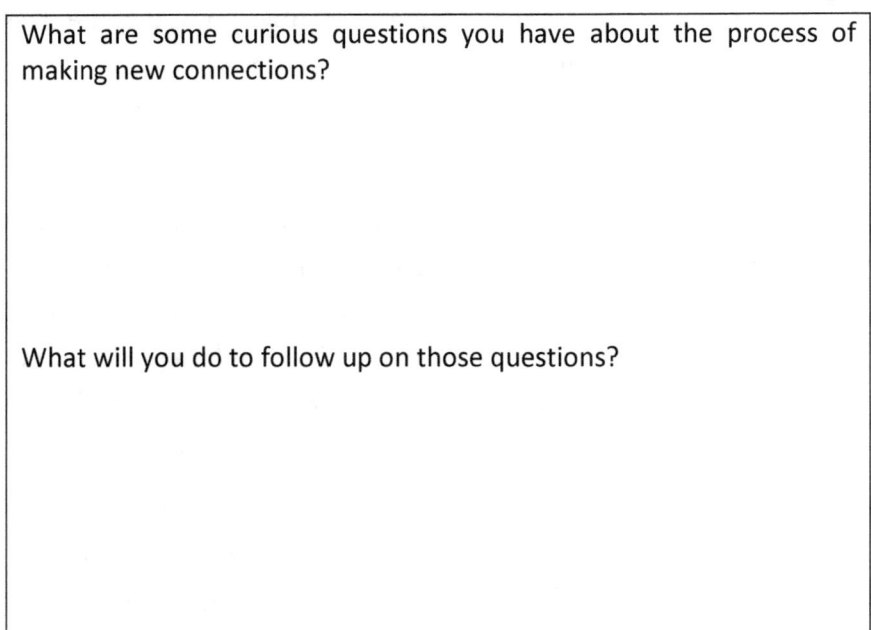

What are some curious questions you have about the process of making new connections?

What will you do to follow up on those questions?

Understand that this process can take time, especially if it's something you haven't done much in the past. Our first friend in Spain was our real estate agent, Antonio, who we met and got to know initially through buying our first apartment in Oviedo in 2022. The three of us (Antonio, my husband Patrick, and I) all liked each other immediately, and we've stayed in touch, having lunch together every few weeks (great for our friendship, and great for Patrick and my Spanish). About a year ago, I told Antonio that I was looking to make other friends locally, but that it hadn't really happened yet. He laughed, and said, *Sucederá–ten paciencia.* ("It will happen–be patient." You can tell he knew me well already.). And he was right; just a year later, I have a handful of good friends and a number of friendly acquaintances. It's definitely heading in the right direction.

Enjoying the Fruits of Your Labors

Once you've made a connection, you need to nourish it. This may also be new to you: many of our connections through work or family get reinforced almost automatically, and don't require a lot of conscious effort.

But in this part of life–and especially with new friends–you'll most likely need to make a bit of effort. It doesn't have to be dramatic; it just needs to be consistent. For example, when we just recently came back to the US for six weeks, I reached out on WhatsApp to each of my four best friends in Spain and told them we'd be back in town by the middle of December and that I'd love to see them during the holiday season. I got lovely responses from each of them, and it felt like a nice little strengthening of our connection.

Think of it as kind of like taking care of houseplants: a little water; a little shift to make sure they're getting enough light; taking off a dead leaf now and then. Just a bit of effort to keep it healthy.

And as for old friends and loved ones...

I don't want to leave this section without touching on your existing connections. I hope you already have people in your life who you love and with whom you have mutually nourishing and beneficial relationships. I probably don't have to tell you how valuable those people are–but it's all too easy to take them for granted. As you focus on making new connections, I encourage you to also think about how to nurture and grow your existing positive connections.

One of my interviewees, a man who has lots of friends and connections old and new, told me recently that he has been putting more attention into strengthening his relationships with his children, who are both in their 30s and living busy lives in cities somewhat distant from him. He noted, "I have a lot more free time than they do, and I realized that I can go and visit them much more easily than they can come and visit me, which is what I was somehow–unfairly–expecting. It's just a matter of being willing to shake up my habit trails a bit. And I was taking their lack of showing up at my house as an indication that they don't care about me, but that's just silly, something I made up. They've been thrilled to have me visit more lately. I'm making the effort to do more FaceTime calls now, too."

So, as you're getting curious about creating new relationships, get curious about how you can deepen and strengthen your most important existing relationships as well. And then–you know what I'm going to say–just do it.

THE BIG IDEA: Connecting with others is key to our health and happiness–and in our third act, as we lose some important connections, we can learn to consciously create new ones.

---

[1] Liebermann, M.D. (2013). *Social: Why our brains are wired to connect.* Crown Publishing

[2] Braren, S. (PhD). (2-24). *The evolution of social connection as a basic human need.* Social Creatures. https://www.thesocialcreatures.org/thecreaturetimes/evolution-of-social-connection

[3] Berg-Weger, M., & Morley, J. E. (2020). Loneliness in old age: An unaddressed health problem. *The journal of nutrition, health & aging, 24,* 243-245. https://link.springer.com/article/10.1007/s12603-020-1323-6

[4] Brown, S. L., & Lin, I. F. (2022). The graying of divorce: A half century of change. *The Journals of Gerontology: Series B, 77*(9), 1710-1720. https://doi.org/10.1093/geronb/gbac057

[5] Escalera, J. (2024) 61% of workers fear retirement more than death, LiveCareer survey finds. LiveCareer. https://www.livecareer.com/resources/retirement-fears

[6] Livingston, G. (2014). *Chapter 2: The demographics of remarriage.* Pew Research Center. https://www.pewresearch.org/social-trends/2014/11/14/chapter-2-the-demographics-of-remarriage/#:~:text=The%20trend%20in%20remarriage%20among,from%20just%2034%25%20in%201960.

[7] Graham, J. (2024, September 14). Historic numbers of older Americans are now living by themselves. *The Washington Post.* https://www.washingtonpost.com/wellness/2024/09/14/seniors-alone-health/

14. And Finally—How It Can Look

"There is a fountain of youth: it is your mind, your talents, the creativity you bring to your life and the lives of people you love. —Sophia Loren

So here we are. Whenever I write a book, I'm talking directly to you, dear reader. I envision you here with me, and I endeavor to share with you those things that I believe will allow you to "crack the code" of whatever challenge the book is meant to help you with; in this case, how to grow old well, and create the life that will be most fun, interesting, satisfying and challenging for you—the life you most want.

Because stories and examples are such a great way to communicate and teach, I always work to incorporate a lot of real-world situations into my books, and I've especially tried to do that with this one, because I've found that positive, realistic stories of older people creating great daily lives for themselves are a little thin on the ground.

You'll notice I've used quite a few anecdotes and stories from my own present life, as I'm definitely working to practice everything I've preached here, and that effort seems to me largely successful at this point. Since those anecdotes have just been glimpses, I thought you might like to get a more complete sense of our life—especially our Spanish adventure—and how that life is fulfilling our visions, my husband's and mine, for this third act.

How it began

When I turned 65, I told my business partners that I wanted to "cut back to full time" at work—and it wasn't really a joke; I was working 50-60 hours a week and wanted to spend closer to 40 hours a week. They were completely supportive, and so we agreed I would work only 4 (10-hour) days a week, instead of 5 or 6, and that I would take more vacation time.

I had also decided to learn Spanish–my book *Be Bad First* had come out the year before, and I wanted to set a big, juicy learning challenge for myself as a way of practicing what I was preaching. Patrick suggested that we vacation in a place where the main language was Spanish so I could practice. As I started researching possibilities, I found myself attracted to the north of Spain; it is greener, more mountainous, and more Celtic than the more popular south. One article described Asturias, in the northwest, as "the Wales of Spain"–and that caught my attention because I have always loved Wales.

So, in 2017, we rented an Airbnb for a couple of weeks near a town called Villaviciosa, and within a few days of arriving, we were–there's no other way to say it–in love with Asturias. Everything about it felt just right to us. The landscape, the people, the food, the culture, the language–everything resonated. We came back in 2018, and then in 2019, we returned again and rented a big house to which we invited our kids, their spouses and our grandkids (of whom there were 3.5 at that point–our younger daughter was pregnant with her first). Everyone had fun and got closer to each other, and our love for Asturias only deepened.

Then came the pandemic...

And everything shifted dramatically. From March to September of 2020, my partners and I focused on pivoting our entire business–coaching, leadership development, and transformation–to virtual delivery. That took up most of my work-attention, and I was also writing my previous book, *Change From the Inside Out*, which seemed both ironic and optimal.

I had a lot of time to walk in the woods, especially during the first few months of the pandemic, when our clients' businesses (and therefore ours) were kind of in suspended animation, and I started thinking more seriously about the next phase of my life, what I wanted it to be like and who I wanted to be as I aged.

By the end of 2021, I had my later-life vision *(In my 70s, I am ELVEN–full of light, deep, strong and magical; my 70s are about EXPLORATION–time to discover, support and enjoy myself, the world, and those I love)*, and our business had survived and was starting to thrive again.

Patrick and I also went back to Asturias when the pandemic restrictions eased at the end of that year, and both of us realized that we wanted to more-than-vacation there; it felt increasingly like an important part of the later life we wanted to create for ourselves. We decided to buy a small apartment in Oviedo, the capital city of Asturias.

At the same time, I realized, as part of my vision, that it was time for me to detach myself even more from Proteus. I told my partners that during 2022, I wanted to step back from managing the company day-to-day, and that by the end of 2023, I wanted to no longer be selling or delivering to clients. We agreed that for 2024 and future years, I would focus primarily on knowledge transfer (getting out of my head key facts and insights about our IP and the process of offering it to clients), sales and marketing communication (including referrals to my network, social media, blogs and our Proteus Leader Show podcast), and advising the senior team. Laird, Jeff, Marie, and I put a lot of energy into figuring out how to do all this in a way that would have the minimum negative impact on the business, the team, me, and them.

Patrick went through a very similar process; he sold his brewery to friends who lived nearby and who already had a very successful farm-to-table wedding business and a fledgling winery, and who wanted to build a tasting room/restaurant on their property. He agreed with them that he would stay on as "brewer emeritus," helping think through new beers and doing other special projects as he and the owner agreed.

As we worked to make that happen, my husband created his own later-life vision. As we spent more time in Oviedo, we both began to realize that it was going to be easier to be who we wanted to be and have the life we envisioned if we spent most of our time in Spain.

So, in 2023, we started the process of applying for long-stay visas in Spain, and we began to think about selling our house in the US. Knowing that we were now only planning on being in the US a few months each year, having to take care of and be responsible for a good-sized house on a big lot out in the country seemed out of sync with the life we were crafting.

I also started writing this book; as Patrick and I worked to bring our visions for ourselves to life, I realized I could also help others craft the lives they wanted in this third act.

We sold our house in the fall of 2024 (a very smooth and non-painful process, thankfully) and rented an apartment closer to New York City. We used the money from the sale to buy a somewhat larger apartment in Oviedo–big enough for our kids and their families, our siblings, or our friends to stay with us when they come to visit–with a big terraza overlooking the city and the mountains.

And now

We're living our vision. When we're in Asturias, my exploration unfolds daily: learning a new language, a new (ancient) culture and city. I'm going to yoga and the gym, taking long walks in the city and the country, enjoying my new friends and taking an open university class on "Myths and Legends of Asturias and Oviedo." Patrick is enjoying life with me, his partner, and finding interesting, unique, useful things to do–his latest obsession is building beautiful rubber-band-powered balsa and tissue-paper model airplanes and flying them in the parks near our apartment. We eat wonderful food, go to great concerts, and enjoy finding out about our adoptive city and its 2,000-year history. We hang out with our friends, both Spanish and expats, and have fun, interesting, wide-ranging conversations.

We're also taking advantage of how easy it is to travel around Europe to lean into the "explore" part of our vision: last year we took trips to Sevilla, Granada and Santiago de Compostela, and this year we've gone to Mallorca, and are planning to visit London or Paris, and perhaps Morocco. We do little day trips to interesting sites in Asturias, too: a milling museum in Taramundi, the Giant Squid museum in Luarca, the 30,000-year-old cave paintings near Ribadesella. Oviedo itself is also full of fascinating stuff–just last week, I spent a few hours in the Museo de Bellas Artes, a five-minute walk from our apartment, simply enjoying the works on exhibit (including Picasso, Joan Miró, and Salvador Dalí).

Technology makes it easy to connect with my colleagues at Proteus wherever I am and to write this book, blog posts, and marketing materials as the team requests.

When we're in the US, we see our siblings and American friends, and we focus most of our time and effort on "discovering, supporting and enjoying" our kids and grandkids (of whom there are now seven) in the various places where they live. We're also exploring our new little city of Peekskill, where our American apartment is, which is interesting and quirky and has a population that's about 45% Latino–a benefit from our point of view both culturally and in our continuing quest to improve our Spanish. Patrick has fun with new brewery projects when we're there (his latest are to create a hydroponic growing system for vegetables outside the tasting room and to explore the possibility of creating a micro-distillery adjacent to the brewing platform).

I do feel full of light, deep, strong, and magical. I can't exactly explain the "magical," but it's there–a sense of ancient beauty and mystery, a kind of sparkling.

I'm sure our lives will continue to evolve in wonderful ways and challenging ways. It isn't perfect: Patrick is dealing with some physical issues, and I've got my "shaky neck," as he so charmingly puts it. But every day, we're grateful for and pleased with the life we're crafting for ourselves, and we know we can continue to do that as we age. We're the boss of our lives, we're mastering our mindset, we're damn good at change, and we're staying connected–with each other and with those we love, family and friends. It's a fascinating adventure...

My Final Gift to You

Before we say goodbye, I wanted to share one last support: a kind of all-in-one doc, where you can put key things to remind you of what you've decided here to support you on this journey of crafting your best later life. You'll find it on the following page and–like all the other activities here–at thenewoldbook.com

Thank you for being on this journey with me, and may you have a wonderful time discovering and creating the third act you truly want.

Be the Boss of Your Life	My Vision:	My strategies (and tactics)
		Qualities I want in my "crew"
Master Your Mindset	My supportive self-talk:	How I stay mindful:
		How I practice gratitude:
Get Good at Change	How I'm managing my mindset about change:	How I recognize when I need to modify:
		What I'll learn next:
How I create and maintain my connections:		

Acknowledgements

So many people have been instrumental in the creation of this book.

First and always, to my darling Patrick. Thank you for being my first reader, my best thinking partner, and the ultimate asker of useful questions.

To Kristi, Kurt and Anne, your support, enthusiasm, and insights have made for a substantially better result–and I'm so grateful that we're family.

To Mom, Dad and David; you left before any of us were ready to have you go. Thank you for being such powerful, honest people; I think of you every day, and your wisdom has found its way onto every page.

To all my interviewees, I so much appreciate your time, thoughtfulness, and humor. Hearing about your challenges and triumphs inspired me and made this a much better book.

To the kids and grandkids: I love you all so much. Hanging out with every one of you is a joy–and I hope we have decades more to grow together.

www.ingramcontent.com/pod-product-compliance
Lightning Source LLC
Chambersburg PA
CBHW061732120626
46550CB00005B/1781

* 9 7 9 8 8 9 5 7 6 0 7 9 6 *